52 Wishes for Walkers

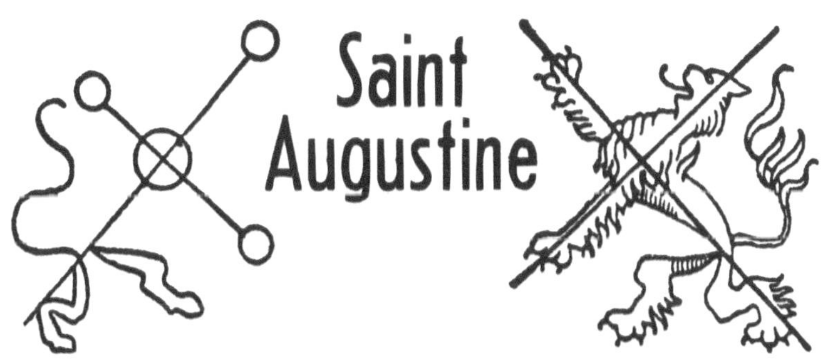

Other titles of interest by Prof. Oddfellow:

How to Be Your Own Cat

A Field Guide to Identifying Unicorns By Sound

Nostradamus Predicted Your Next Diet

How to Believe in Your Elf

Strange Prayers for Strange Times

Seance Parlor Feng Shui

The Young Wizard's Hexopedia

One-Letter Words: A Dictionary

For the spirited guide
Gordon Meyer ...

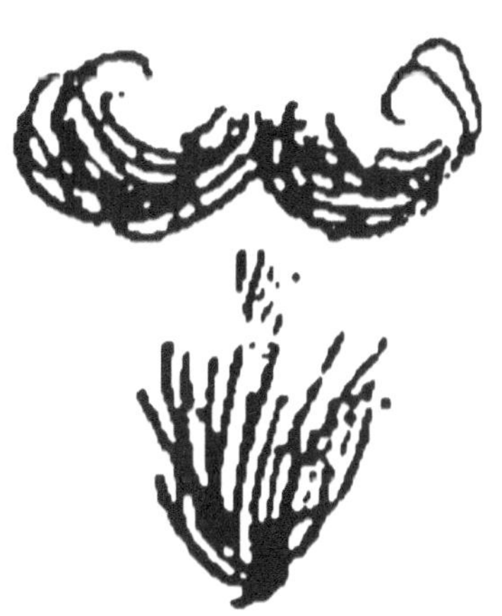

who walked back in time
to be in *Le Journal Amusant*, 1905.

Whoever
knows this book
shall go out into the day,
shall walk among the living
and shall never suffer destruction.
This fact is a million times authentic.
—*The Egyptian Book of Going Forth By Day*

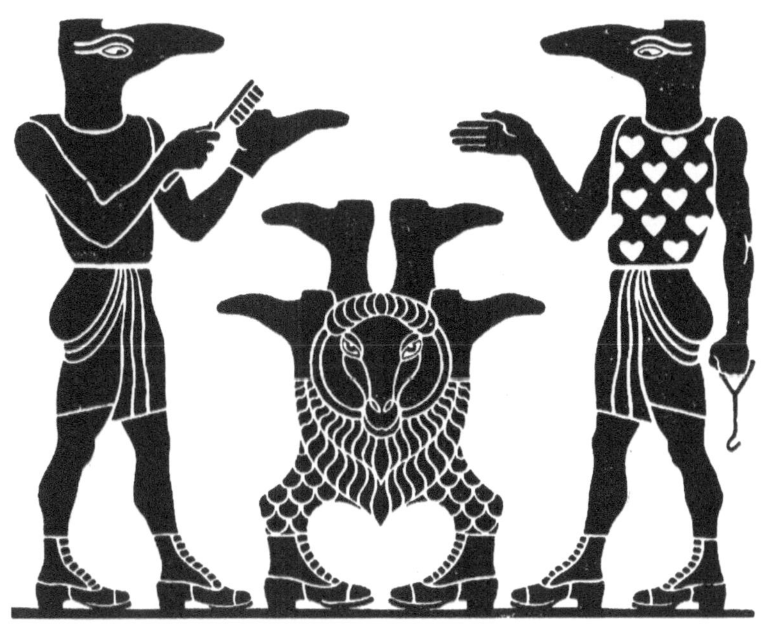

[These spirit guardians of walkers appeared in a
shoemaker's advertisement in *Jugend* magazine, 1898.]

Introduction:

Why a Journey
Does *Not* Actually
Begin with a Single Step

It's commonly said that a journey begins with a single step. But what motivates that step?

* an itinerary
* a destination
* a conscious plan
* a sense of purpose
* the seed of an idea
* opening one's heart
  to brand new possibilities

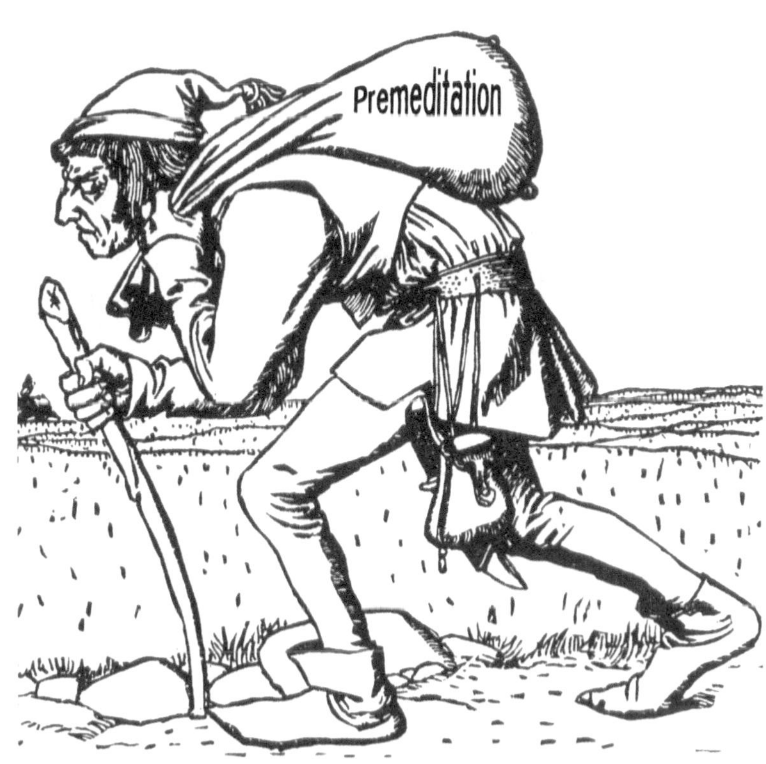

And so collected herein are 52 wishes for wayfarers
before they take that first step, one for every bone
of the feet. Some might be called blessings, others
prayers and positive affirmations for those who would
travel by foot. There is even a trio of ancient foot
talismans from the Far East.

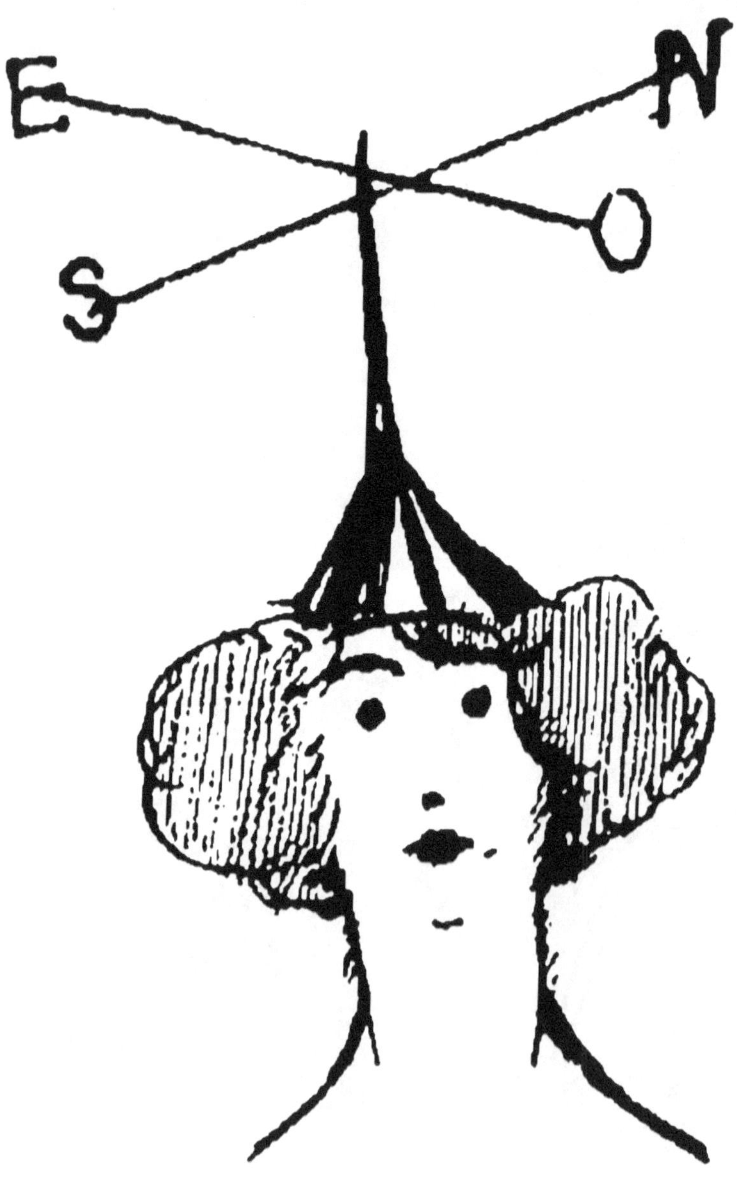

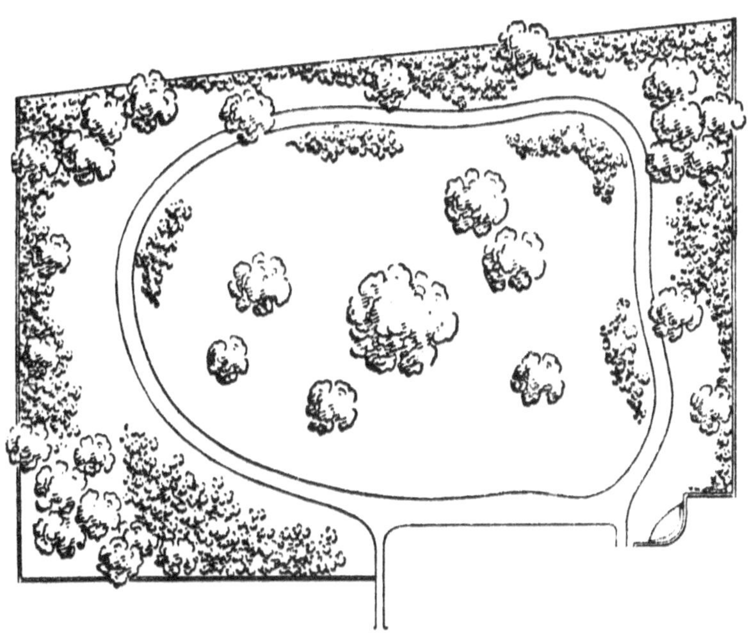

May you walk your path with curiosity, delight, and
intention.
—Elizabeth Murray, *Living Life in Full Bloom*

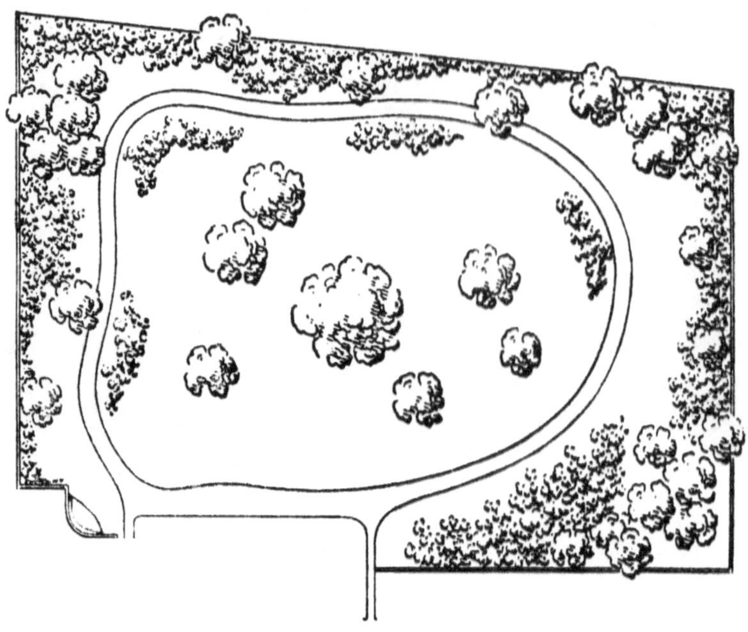

May you go forth
having power over your feet in the morning,
having power over your feet by torchlight,
having power over your feet at all times
and at any hour you wish to go forth.
—A prayerful spell from the ancient *Pyramid Texts*,
reproduced in *Death and Salvation in Ancient Egypt*
by Jan Assmann

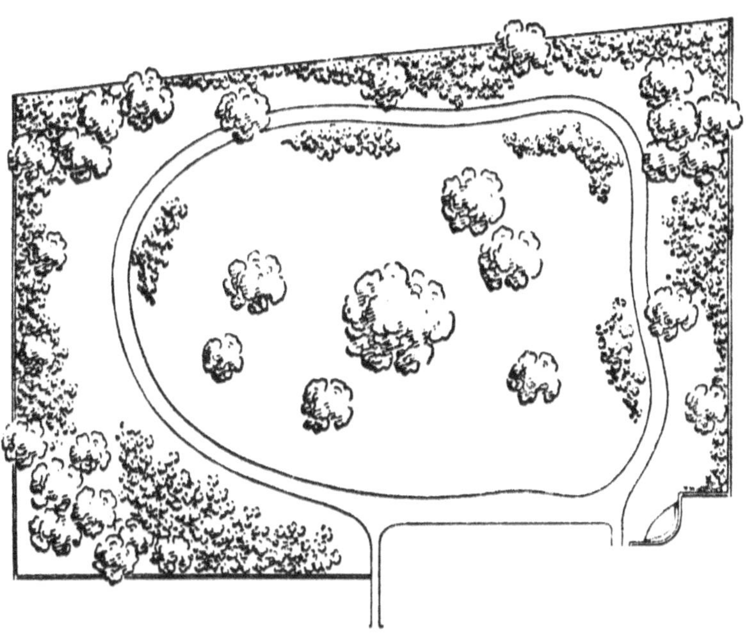

May your tour be fruitful in that it gives you the opportunity to see with your own eyes real life in this country.
—*Foreign Affairs Bulletin*

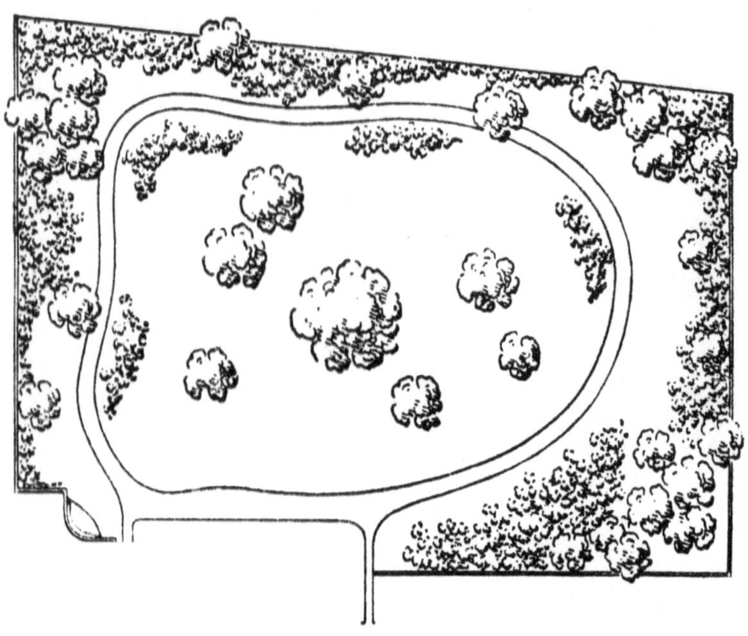

Step by step, may you be rewarded.
—Camilo Gómez-Rivas

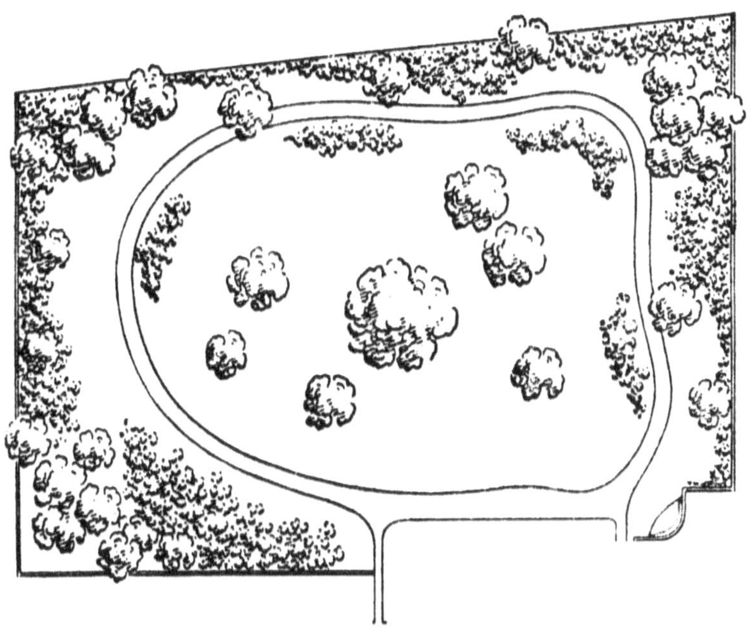

Let yourself be led gently along the path of your own becoming.
—Phil Small, *On the Way to Here*

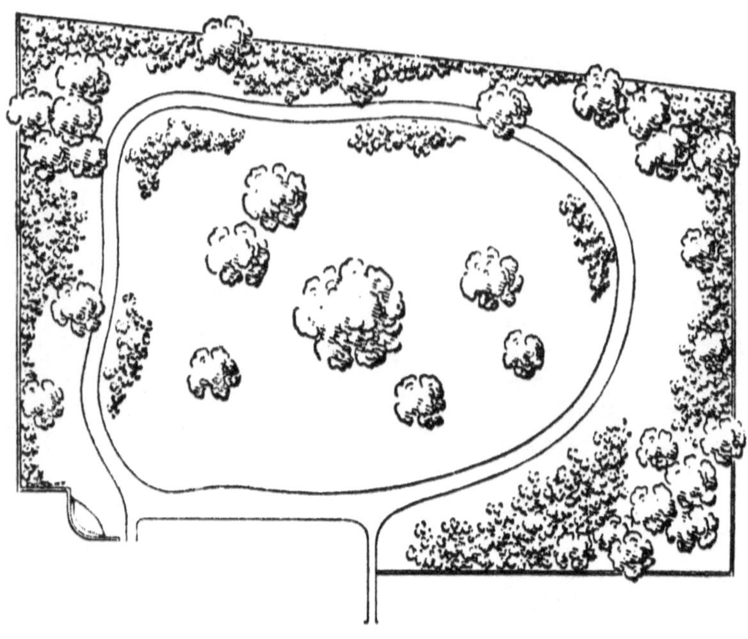

Let your feet be *knowing-something* feet.
—Gabriel Okara, "Birth Dance of the Child-Front"

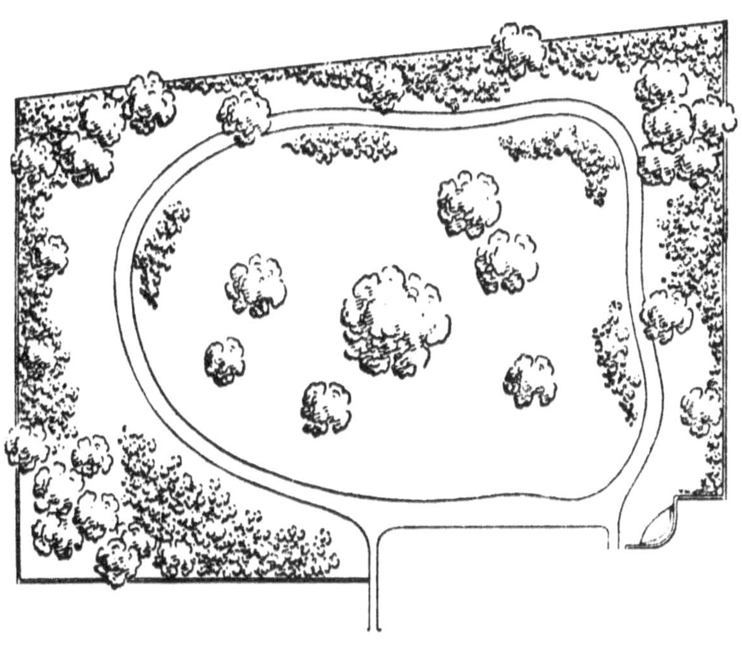

The soles of your feet are firm every day;
your toes guide you on fair paths.
—*The Egyptian Book of Going Forth By Day*

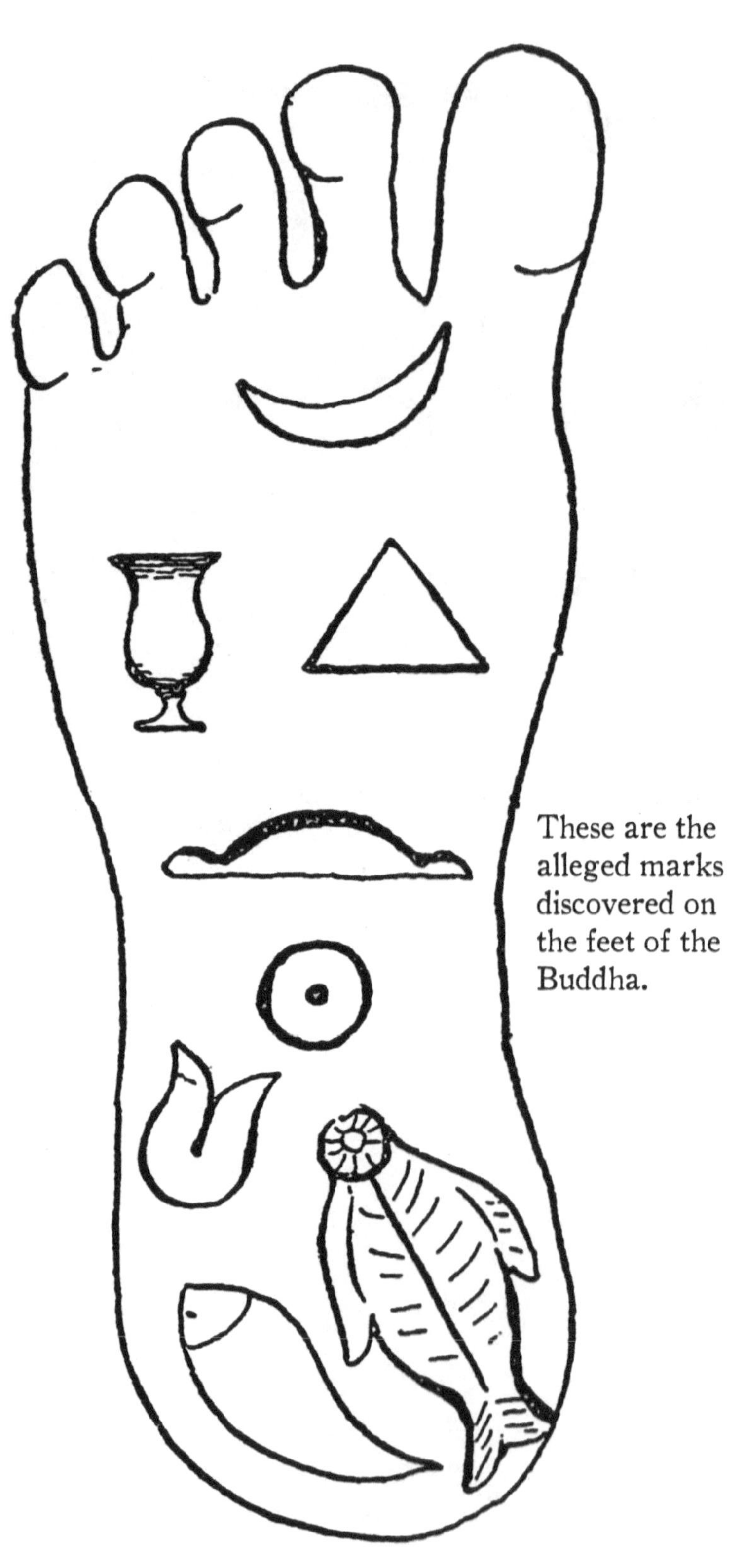

These are the
alleged marks
discovered on
the feet of the
Buddha.

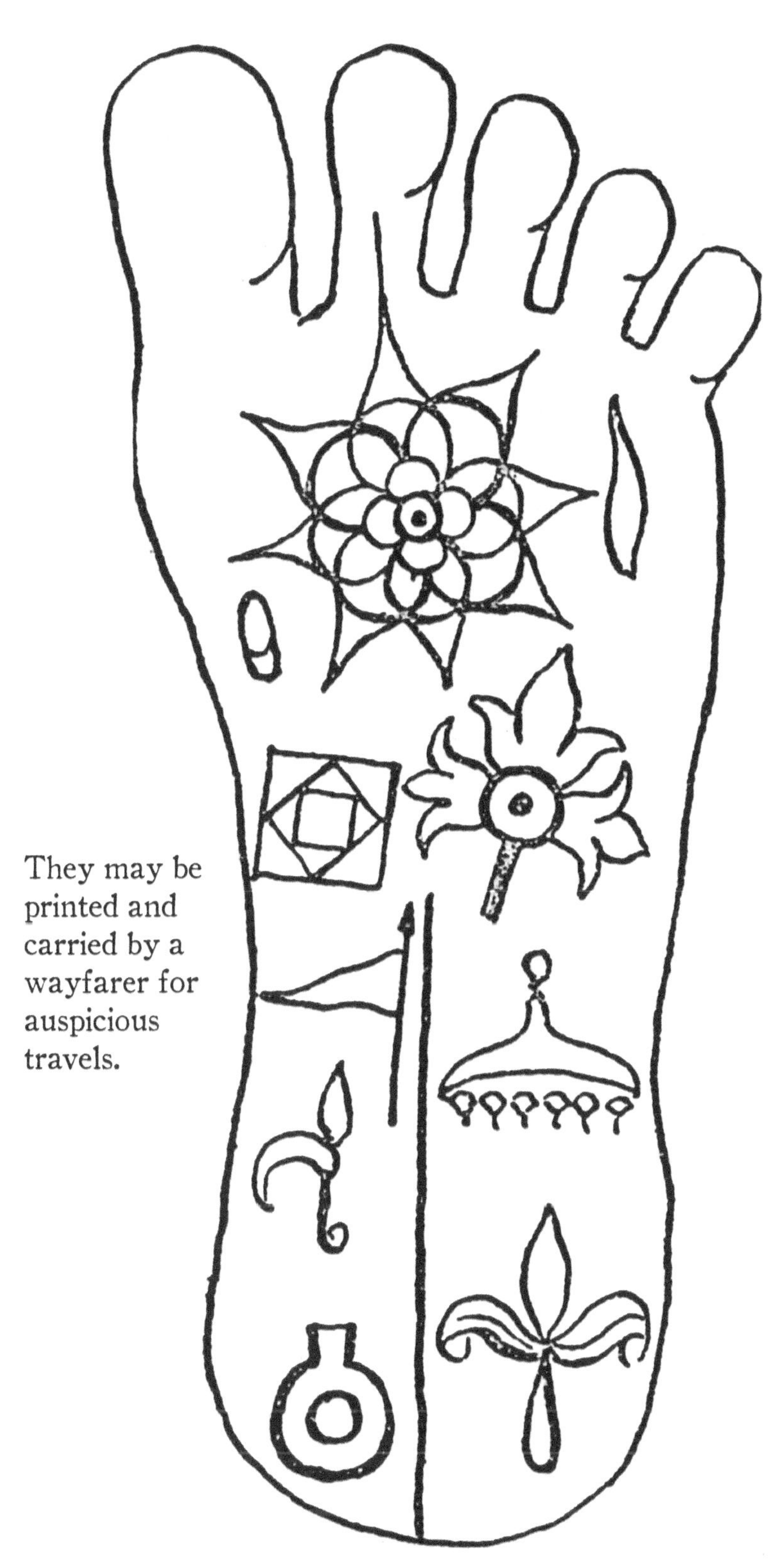

They may be
printed and
carried by a
wayfarer for
auspicious
travels.

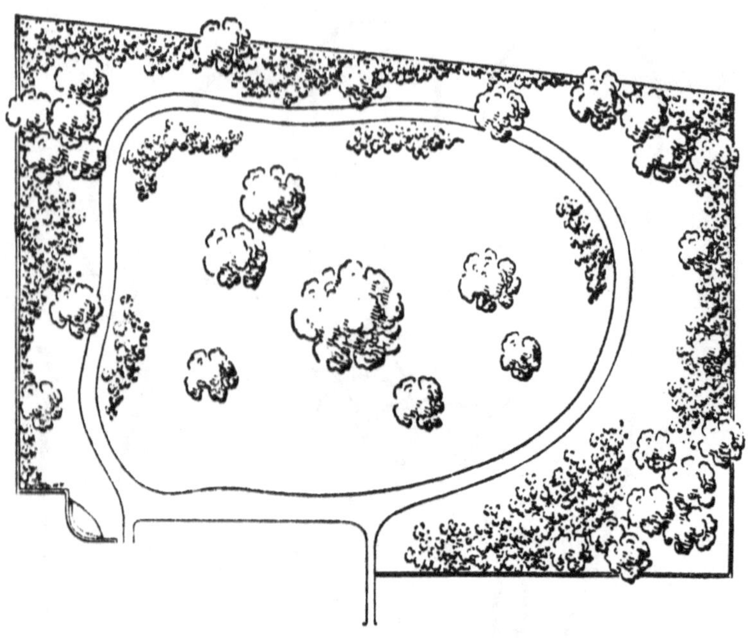

May your feet carry you along the path.
—Naomi Kritzer, *Fires of the Faithful*

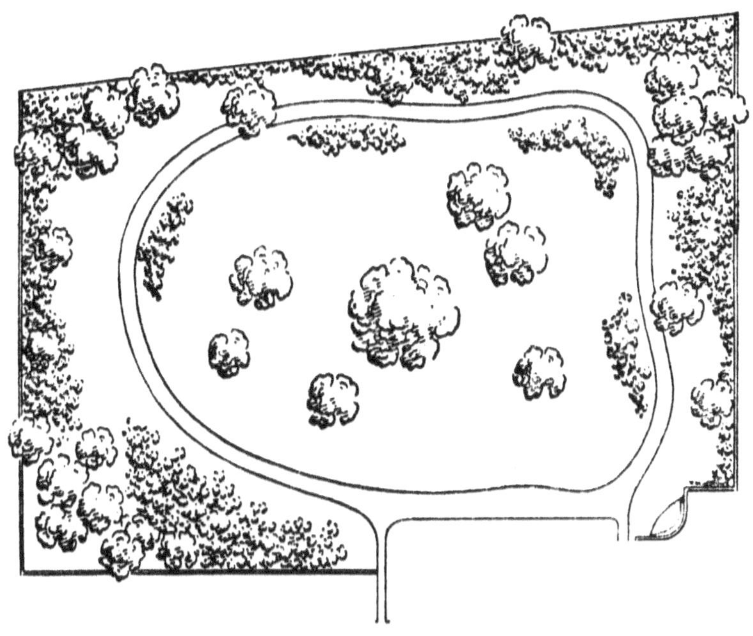

May each step of your journey be filled with love.
—Lynn A. Anderson, *The Nectar of Love*

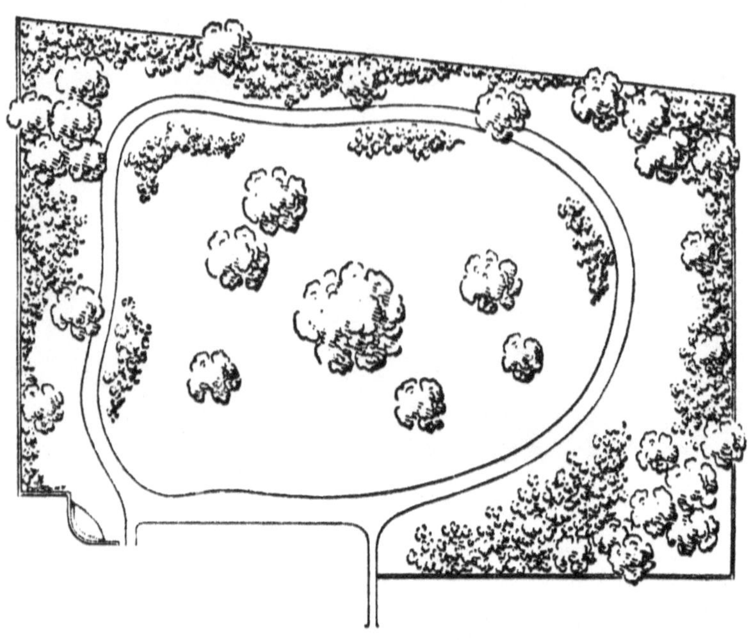

May your feet be up to the task.
—Ovid, *Remedia Amoris*

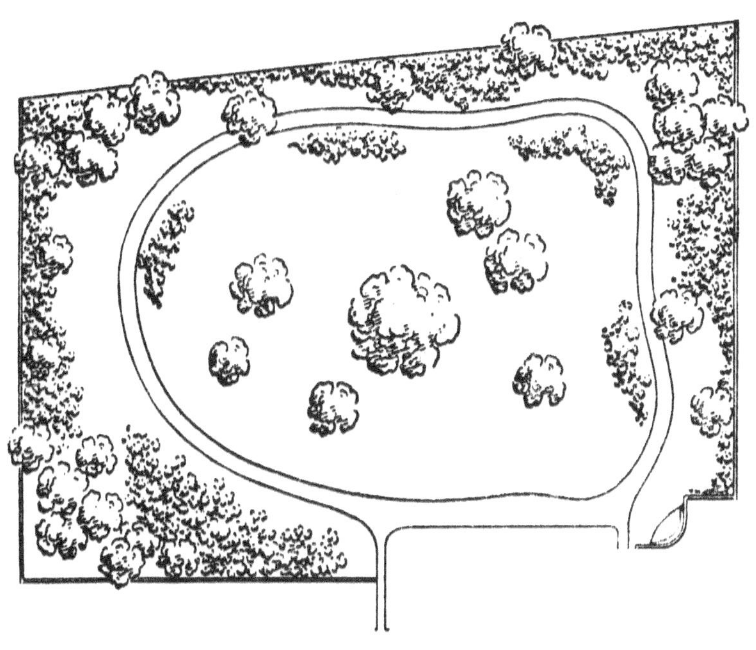

Let your every step be forward.
—*Everybody's Poultry Magazine*

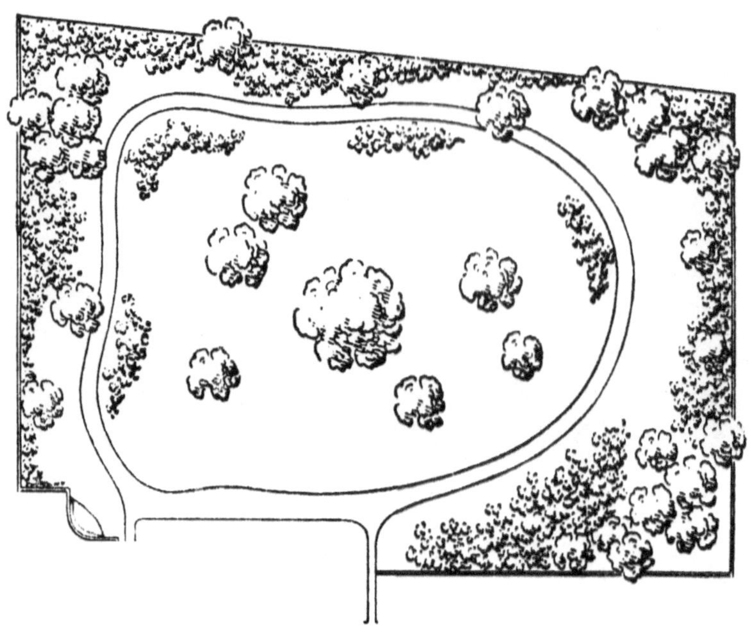

May your feet carry you safely home.
—*The Epic of Gilgamesh*

The legendary Chinese Emperor Yu of the Xia dynasty created his own system of mystical footwork based upon the arrangement of the constellations as well as mimicry of the movements and dances of the animal kingdom. Yu's steps were intended to establish harmonic balance both within the human microcosm and outward into the universe. His complex choreographies gave birth to the modern steps of Tai Chi, Kung Fu, and other martial arts.

Diagrams of Yu's footwork, handed down through the ages, serve as talismans for making the right moves in life. The first talisman here reproduced shows a spiral pathway for circulating the bodily energies and centering oneself. The second talisman shows Yu's dance entitled "Pace the Big Dipper," for symbolically bringing the celestial order down to earth and acquiring astral lucidity.

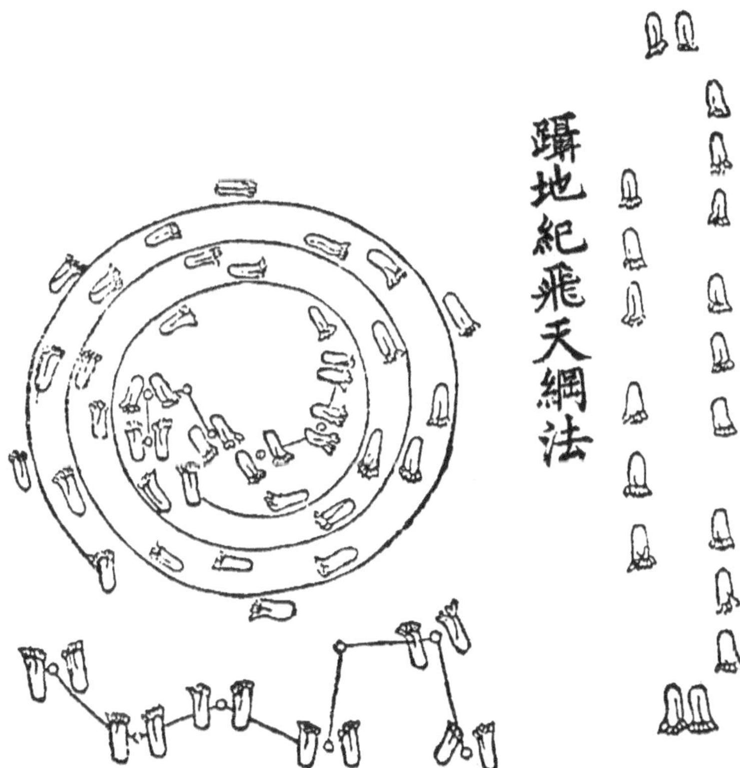

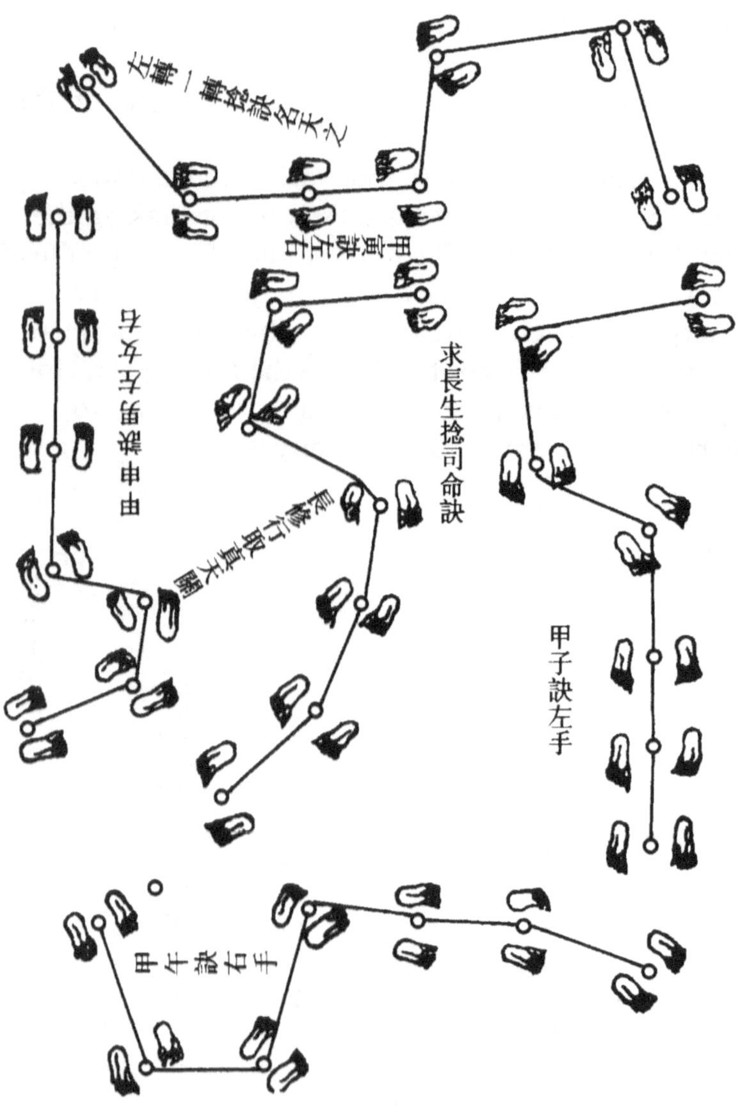

左轉
轉捻巷名天之
甲寅訣左右
求長生捻司命訣
長檢行取真天關
由申子牙
甲子訣左手
甲午訣右手

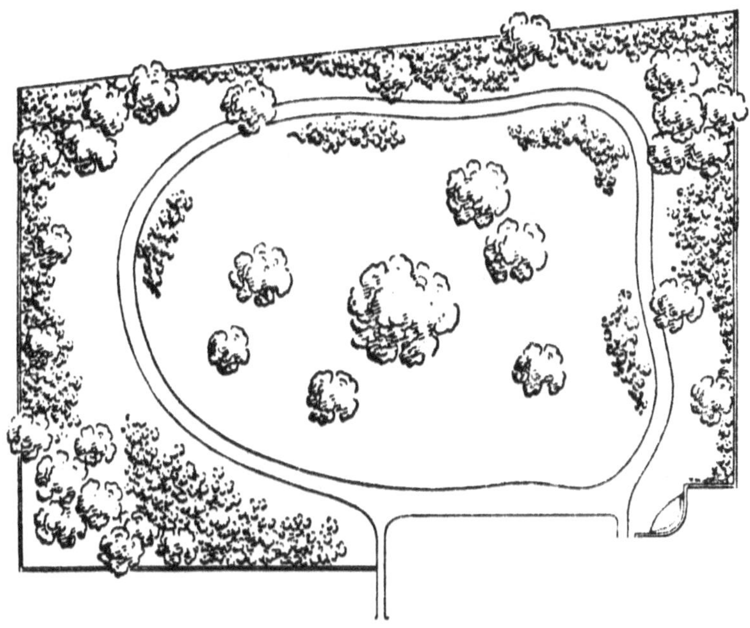

May you walk through life with *Shechina* [the divine presence] guiding you, guiding you.
—Myrna Rabinowitz, "A Blessing for My Daughter"

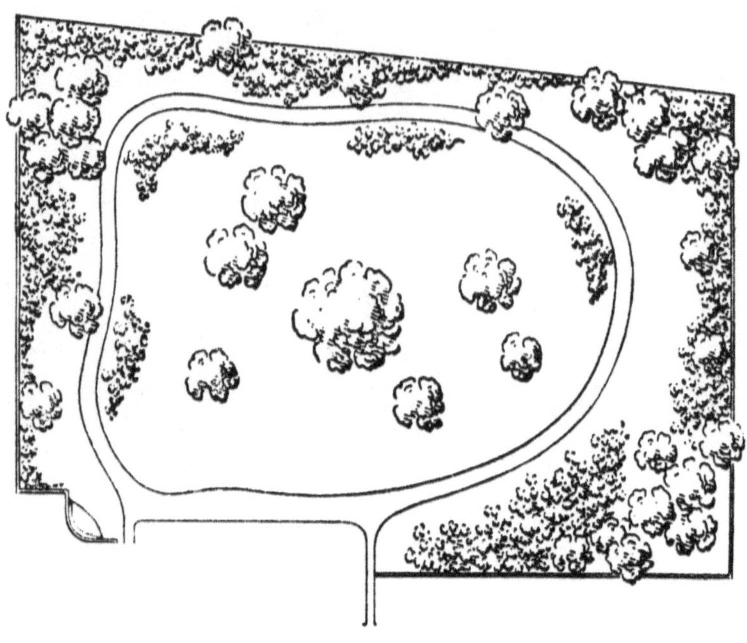

May you walk in beauty in a sacred way.
—From a Sufi song, reproduced in *The Experience of Divine Guidance* by Mark Allan Kaplan

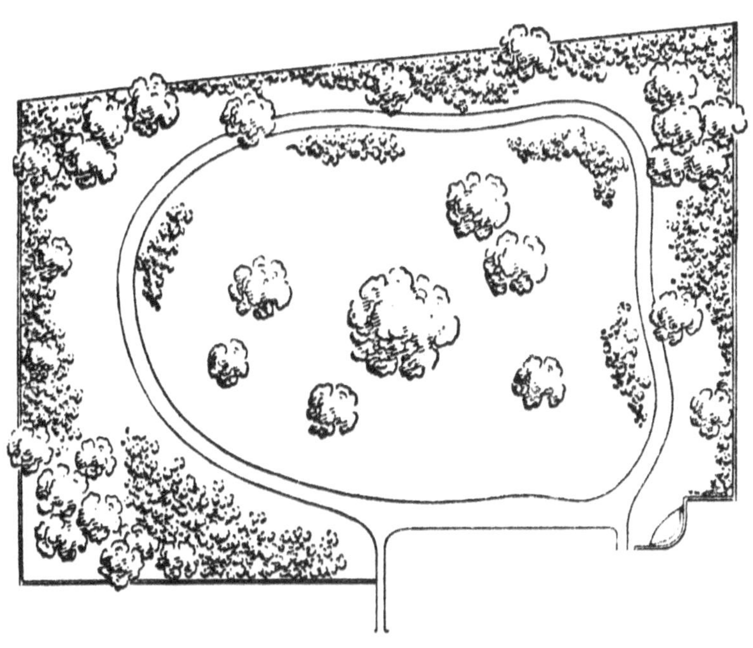

I shall go out into the day,
I shall walk on my feet,
I shall have power in my strides.
—*The Egyptian Book of Going Forth By Day*

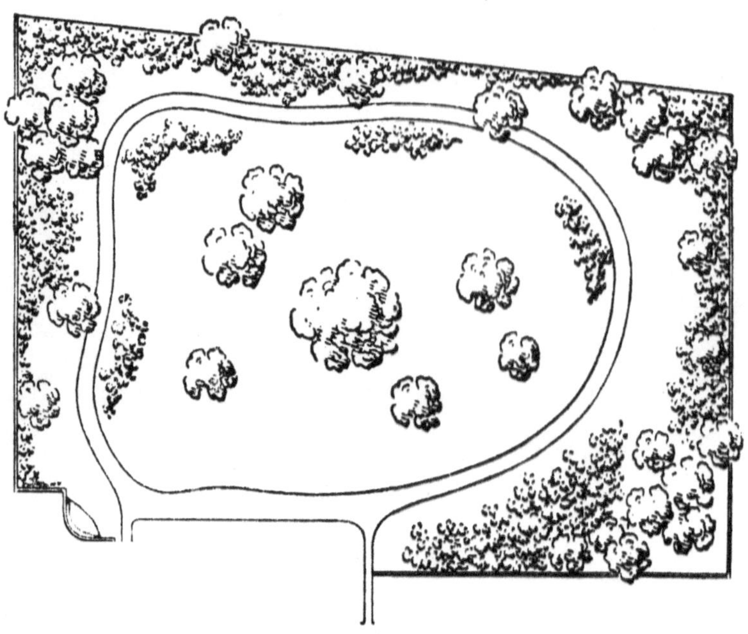

May your feet always be swift.
—Bob Dylan, "Forever Young"

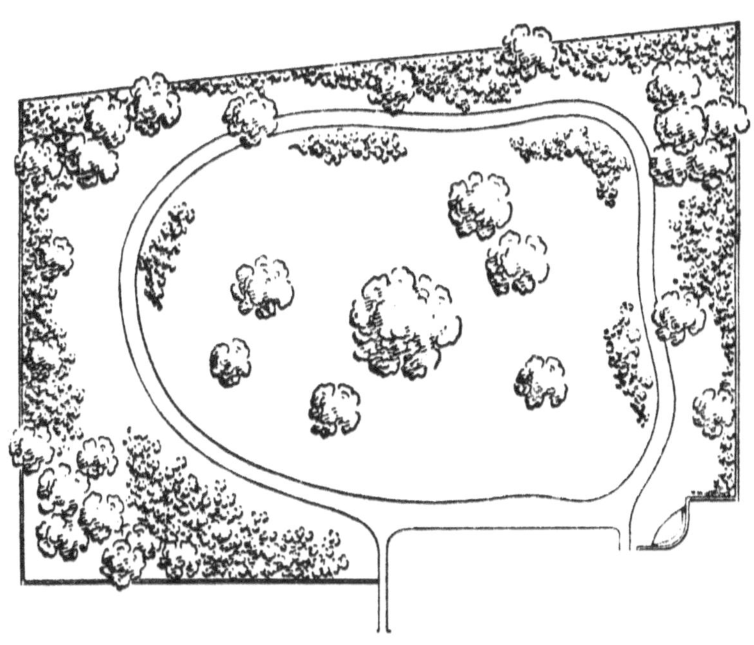

Mantra for blessing the feet:
Om khrecha raghana hum hri svaha
[Recite this mantra three or seven times and spit on
the soles of your feet or shoes. Then any insect that
dies under your feet during the day will be born
in the Thirty-three deva realm. This is from the
Manjugosha Root Tantra.]
—Lama Zopa Rinpoche, *Bodhisattva Attitude*

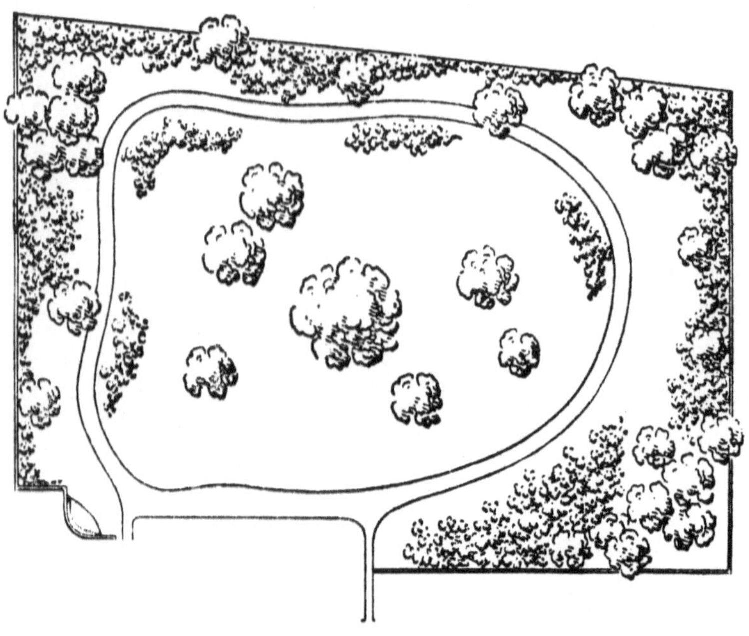

May you walk on silver ground and a floor of gold.
—*The Egyptian Coffin Texts*

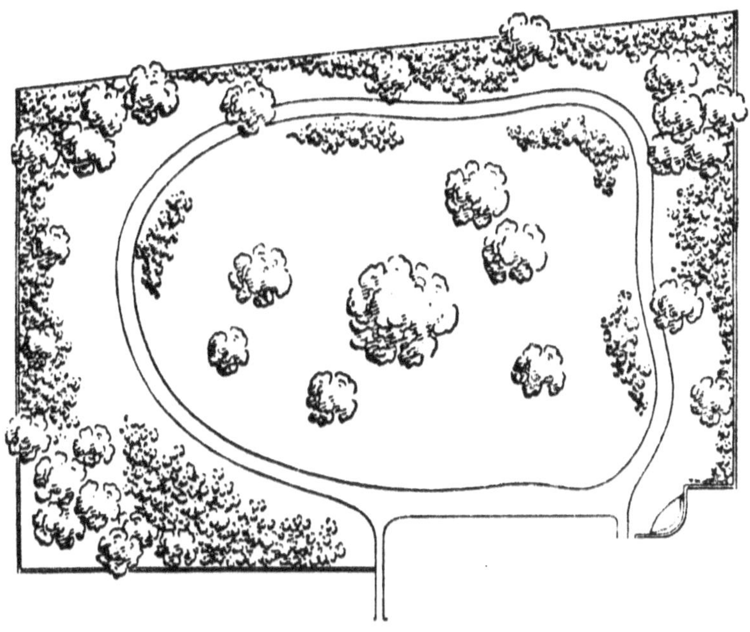

I pray that your feet may not depart from the ways
of wisdom.
—William J. Kerby

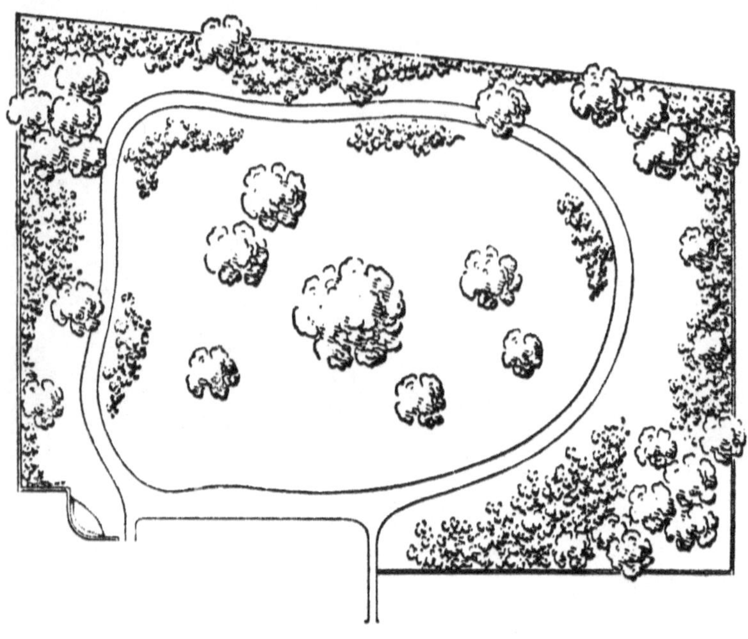

With each step may the mystery of life unfold.
—Curtis E. Crawford

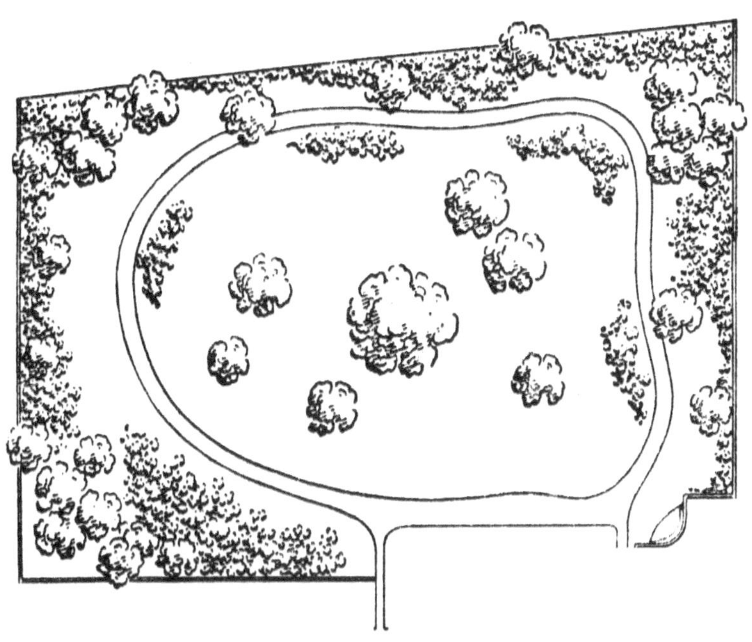

May each step you take be easy ...
May the road you travel be easy.
—Darryl Barnett, *A River of Dreams*

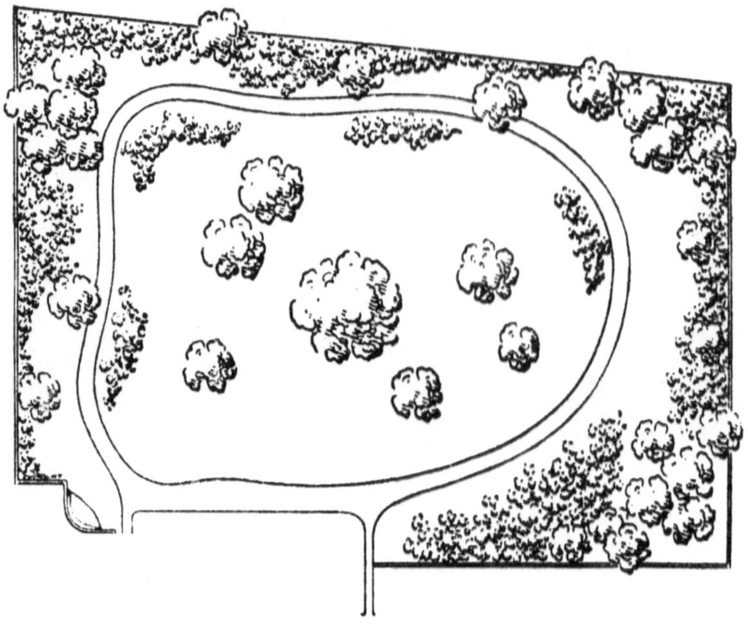

May your feet always find the paths to the Sacred
Grove.
—Sara Douglass, *Starman*

May St. Christopher, holy patron of travelers, protect you and lead you safely to your destiny.
—A traditional prayer

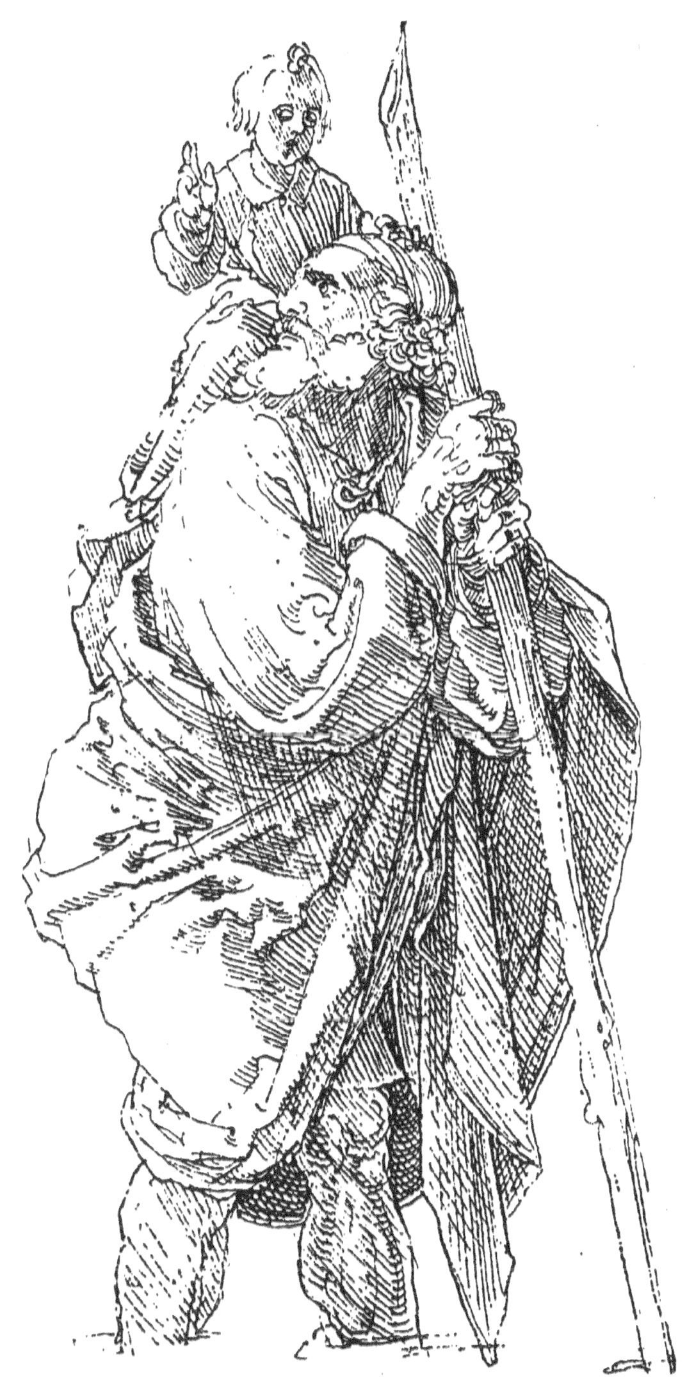

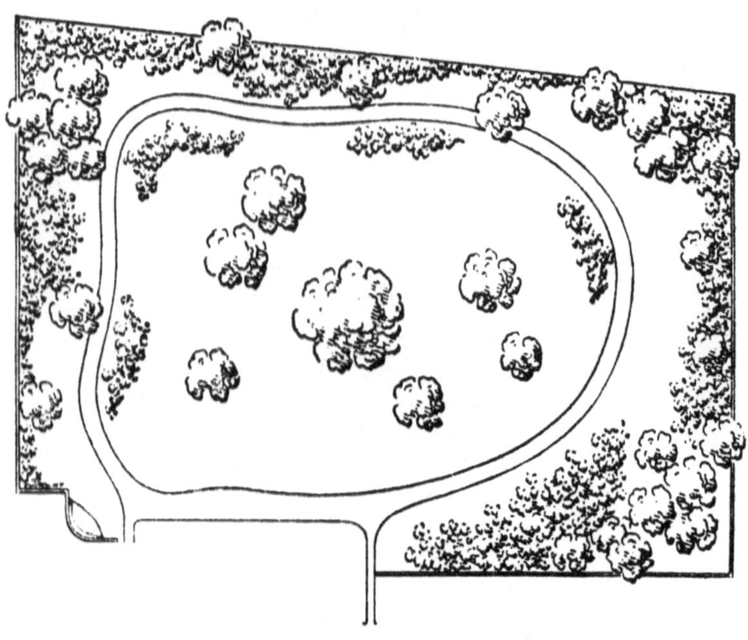

May your every journey be a happy one.
—Marie Gozzaldi

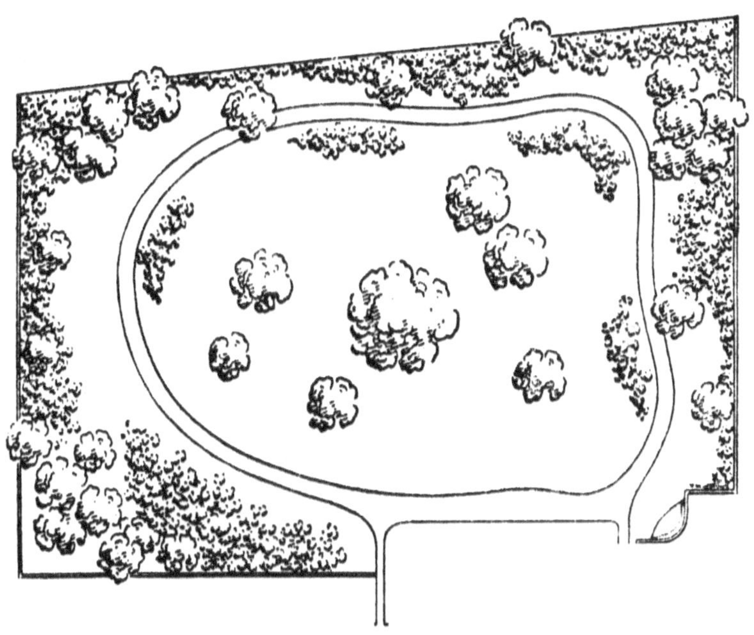

May the earth welcome your footsteps,
May the wind sing your tale.
—From a blessing song by Raven Kaldera

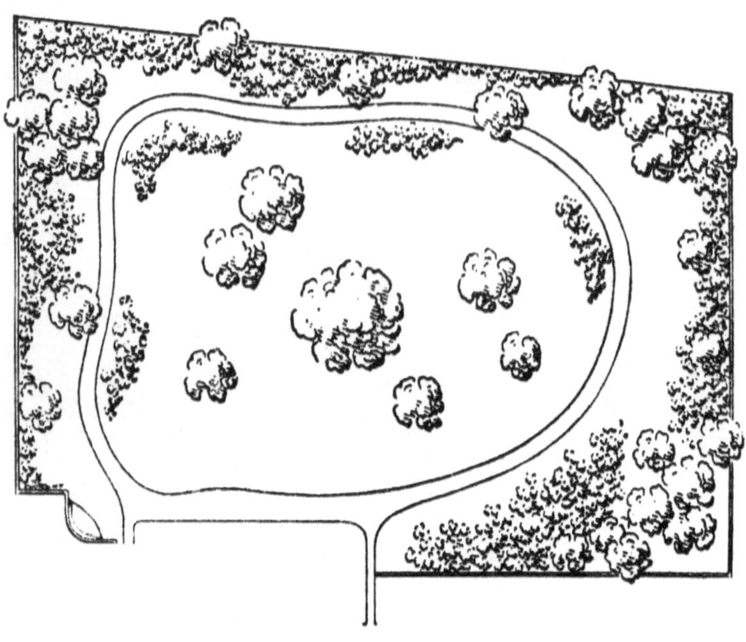

May your journey be fruitful.
—Calvin Cassady, *Bridging the Gap*

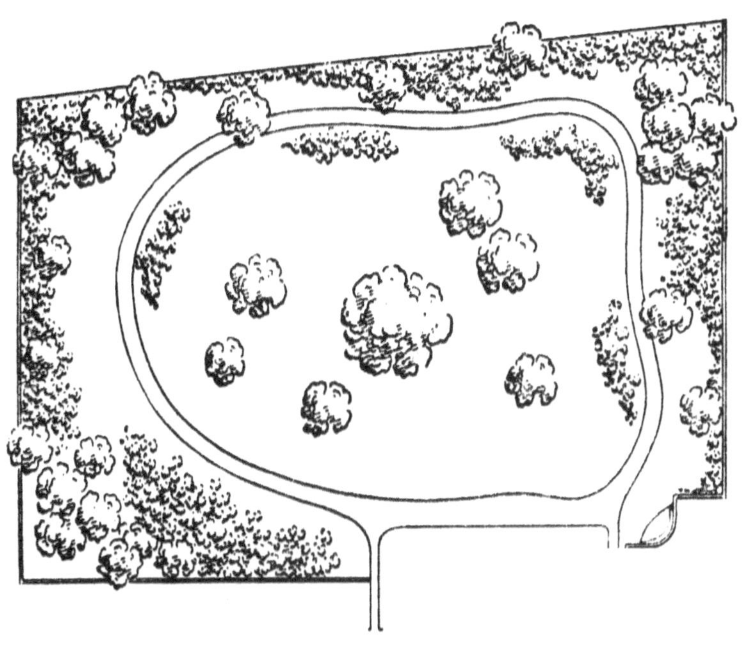

May your feet be blessed.
—Julieanne Lynch, *In the Shadows*

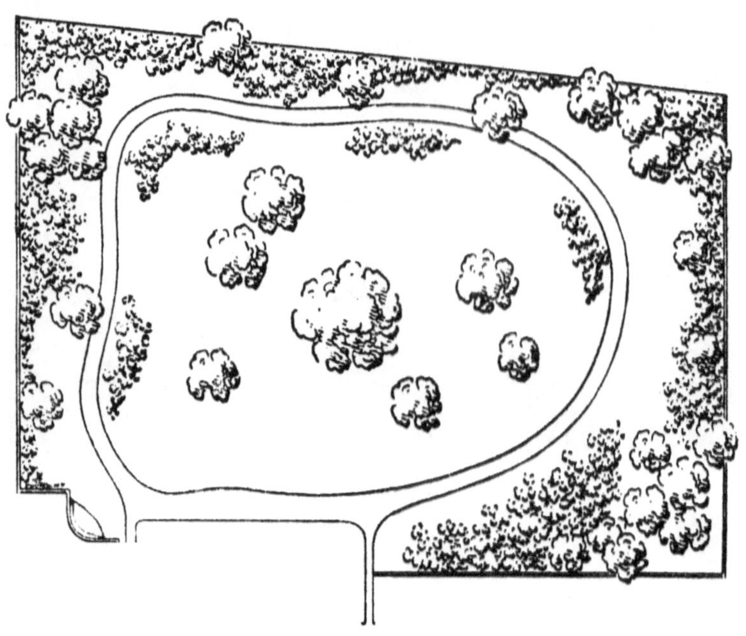

May you not walk head downward.
—*The Egyptian Book of Going Forth By Day*

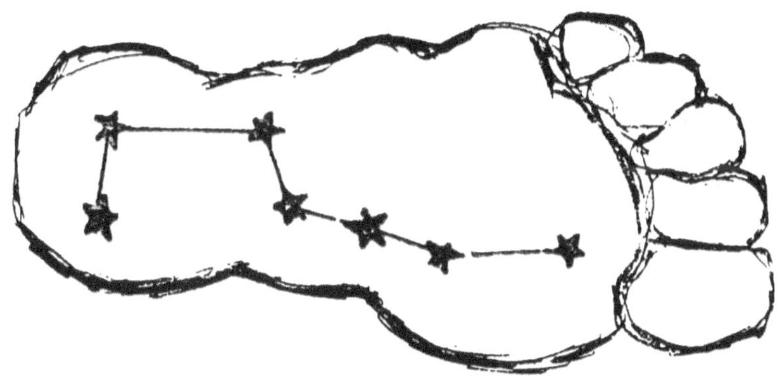

In Taoism, respect is paid to the seven stars of the Big
Dipper constellation as a way of transforming one's
negative luck into positive luck and of prolonging
one's lifespan. A magical charm is created by printing
onto red paper diagrams of the feet with Big Dippers
on the soles. These diagrams are stood upon while
one pronounces an incantation, each foot completely
covering the stars in the constellations:

Move cautiously on!
O ferns, o ferns, wound not my steps!
Through my tortuous journey, wound not my feet!
The Big Dipper of the Open Valley is divine
and so it can dispel the devils.
Quickly, quickly,
in accordance with
the statues and ordinances.
Act, as this is my command.

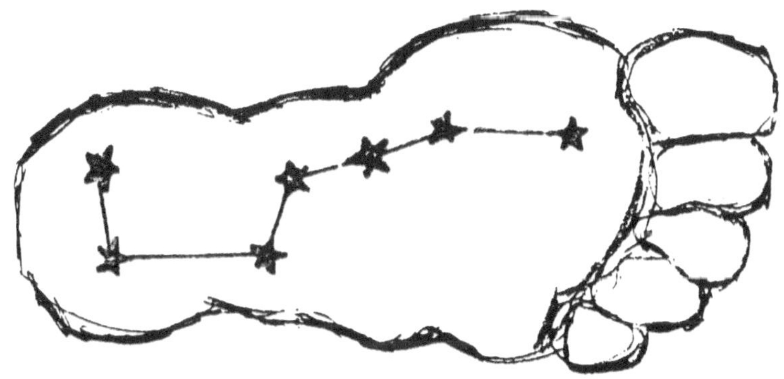

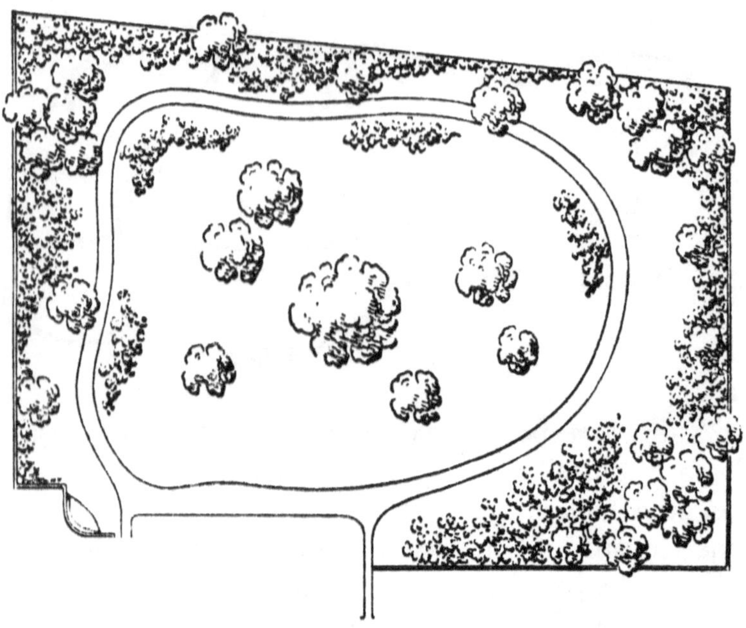

May your feet rest for a long time on the ground.
—A wish upon wearing buffalo-hide moccasins for
the first time, spoken while turning around four times,
in Stephen D. Peet's *Myths and Symbols*

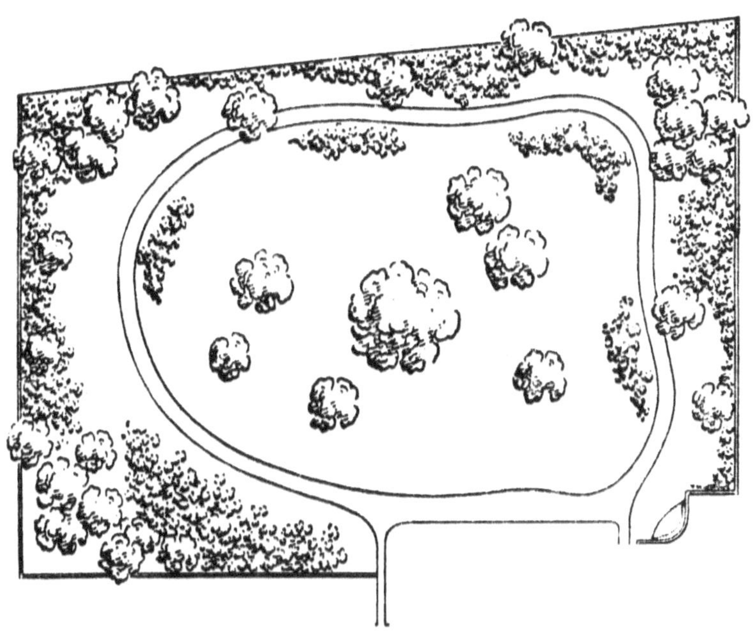

I pray that your journey will always be one of awe.
—Cynthia Heald

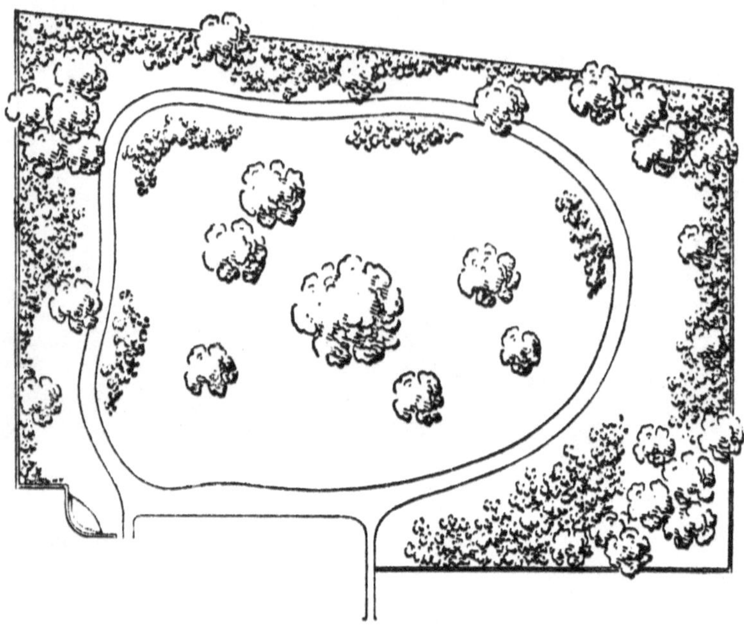

May you walk away content, satisfied with the sound
of your own answers.
—Mary Anne Radmacher, *Us!: Celebrating the Power
of Friendship*

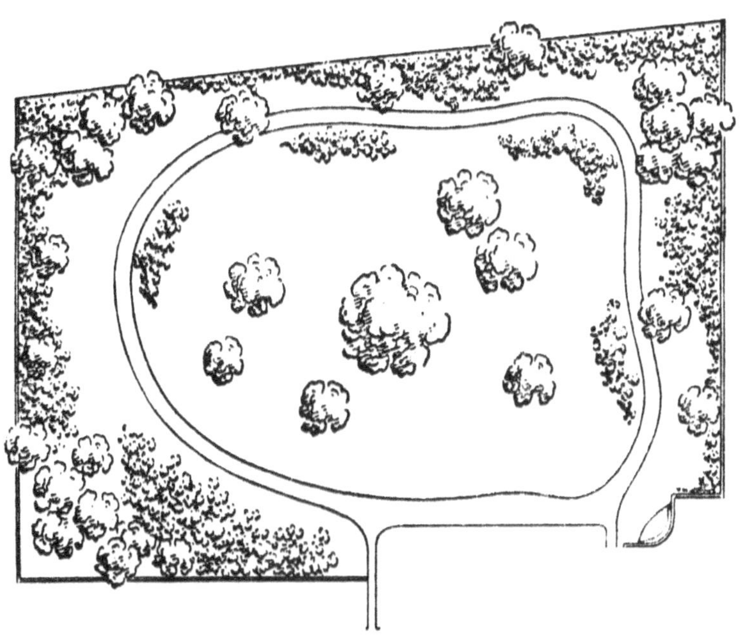

May your soul be free ...
May your eyes see only beauty ...
May your strides be swift ...
May your feet take you there.
—Wayne O. Holness, *Sherroll*

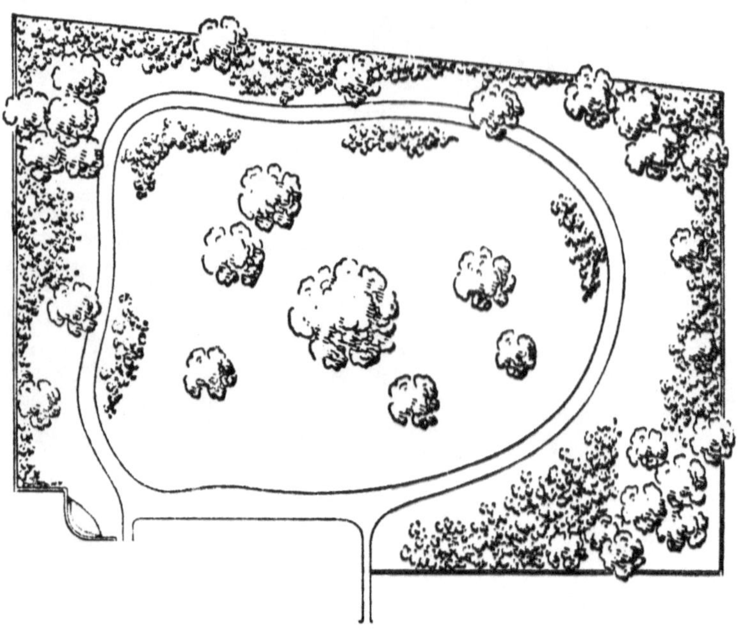

May you walk in prosperity.
—*The Teahouse of the August Moon*

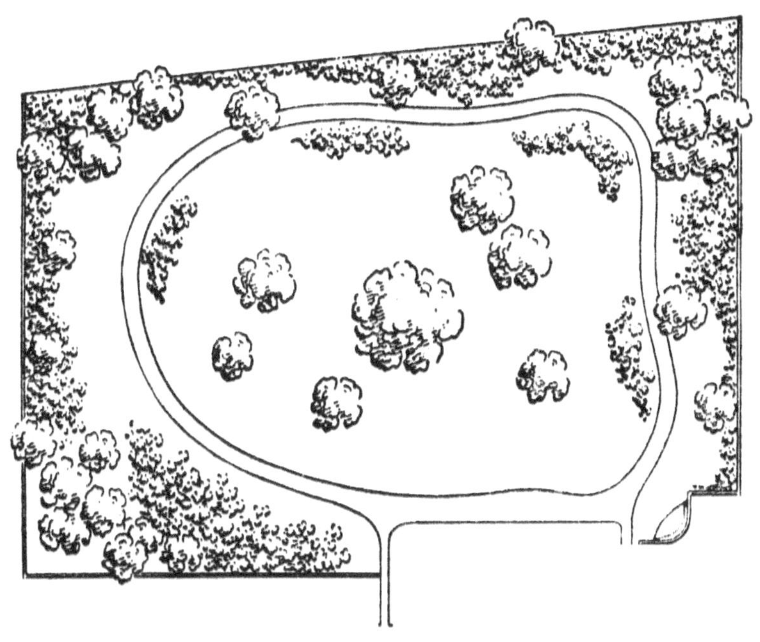

My wish is that you take that first step.
—Harmony Rose

May every step we take be a step in the right
direction.
—Joseph Parker, *These Sayings of Mine*

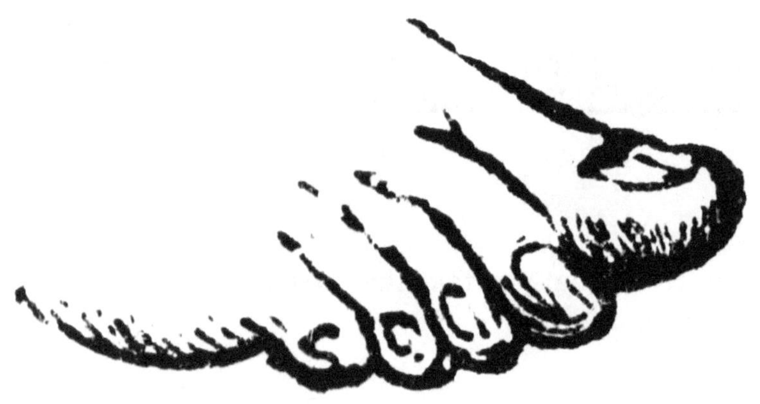

Did you know that the toes are aligned to the
five norths?

The big toe: True North
The second toe: Magnetic North
The third toe: Celestial or Astronomical North
The fourth toe: Grid North
The fifth toe: Terrestrial North

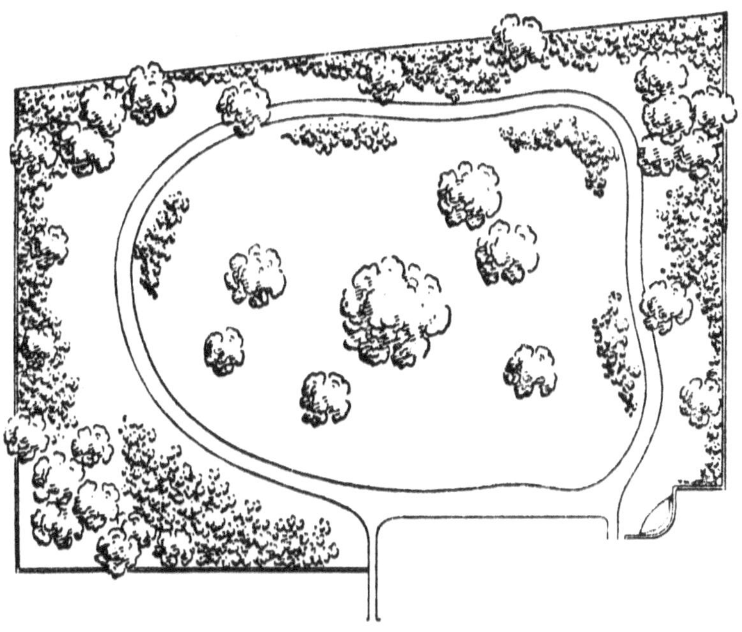

May you walk with sunlight shining
And a blue bird in every tree.
—Meredith Wilson, "May the Good Lord Bless and
Keep You"

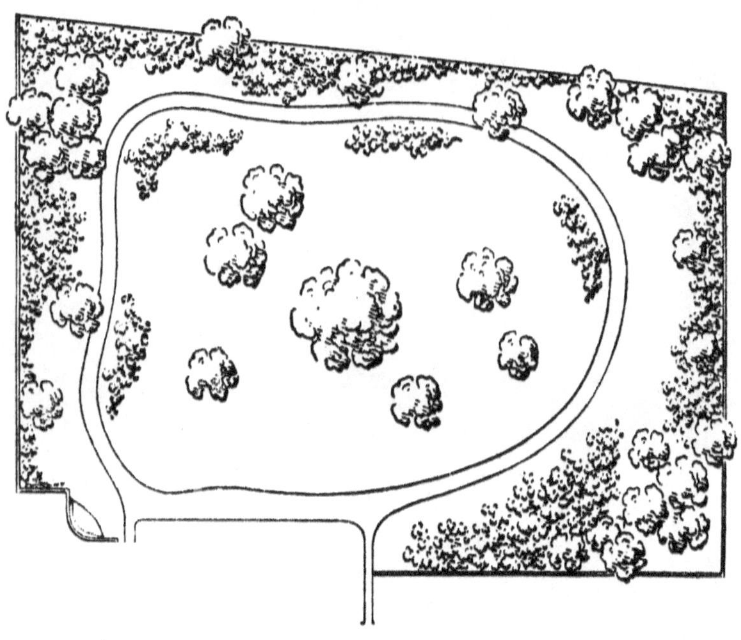

May your path be ever upward.
—George Everard, *Your Sundays*

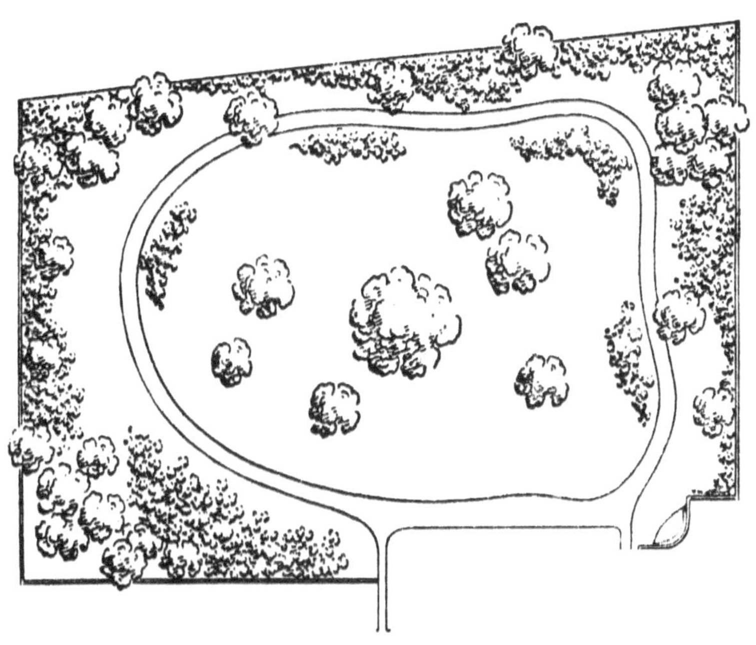

May the life of ye be long
And the death of ye be aisy;
And may each of your toes
Give birth to a daisy.
—A traditional wish reproduced in *The Pittsburgh Sun*

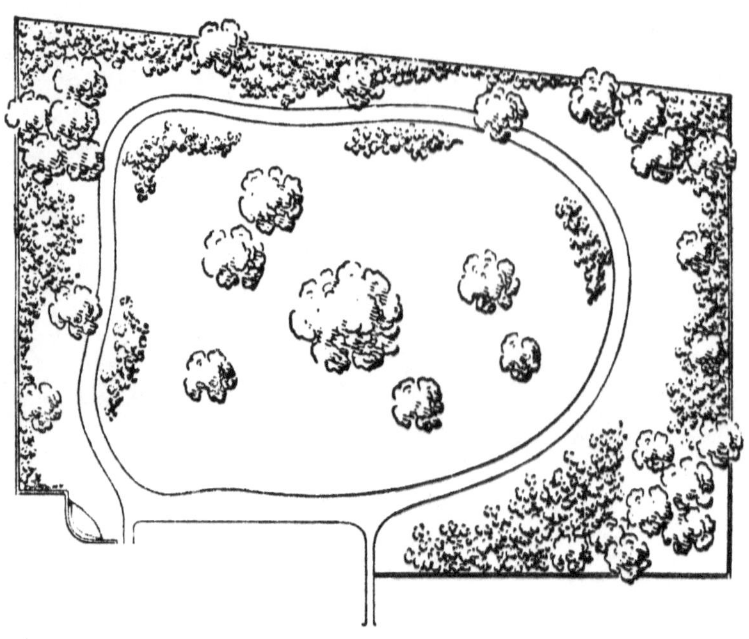

May you walk the trail of beauty.
—Glenn Dixon, *Pilgrim in the Palace of Words*

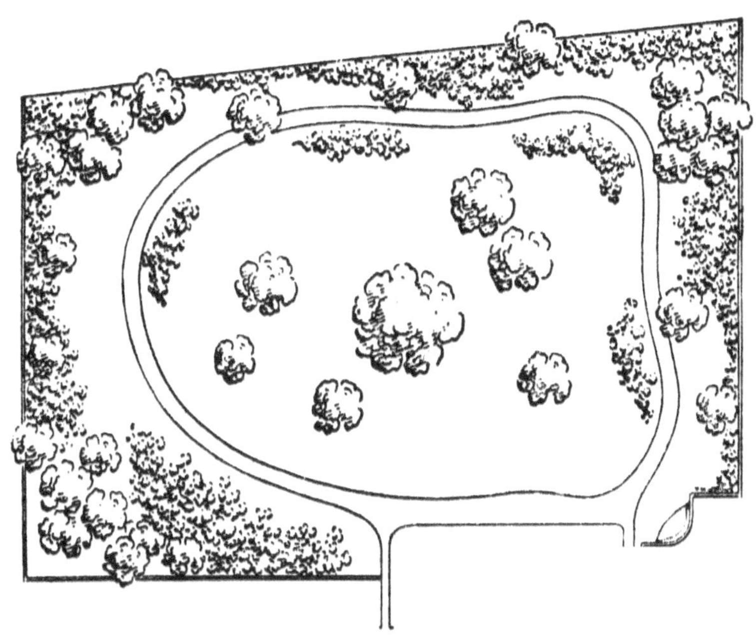

Whenever you journey, may your steps be firm and
may you walk in just paths and not be afraid.
—Rabbi Sandy Eisenberg Sasso, "Parent's Prayer"

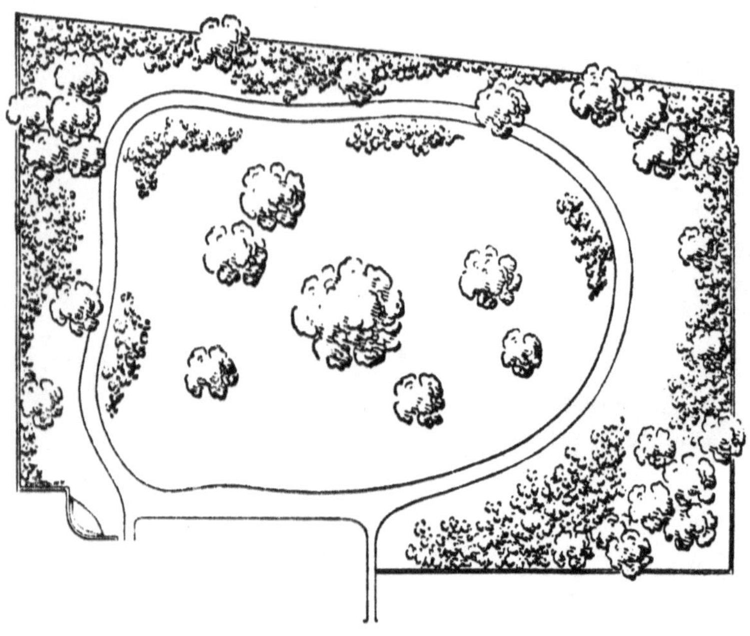

May your steps be always sure.
—*The Very Best of Paul Cookson*

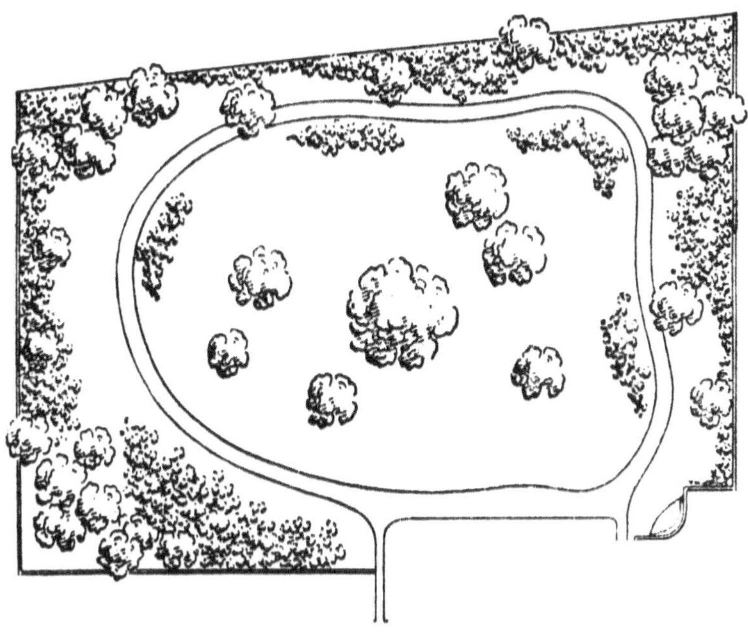

May every journey through the past remain imbued
with a little humility and respect for the mystery of
time, and each visit be like a tau that we mark on
our own stone, the stone that each of us is destined to
become in the wall of human history.
—Andrew White, *Time Out Book of Paris Walks*

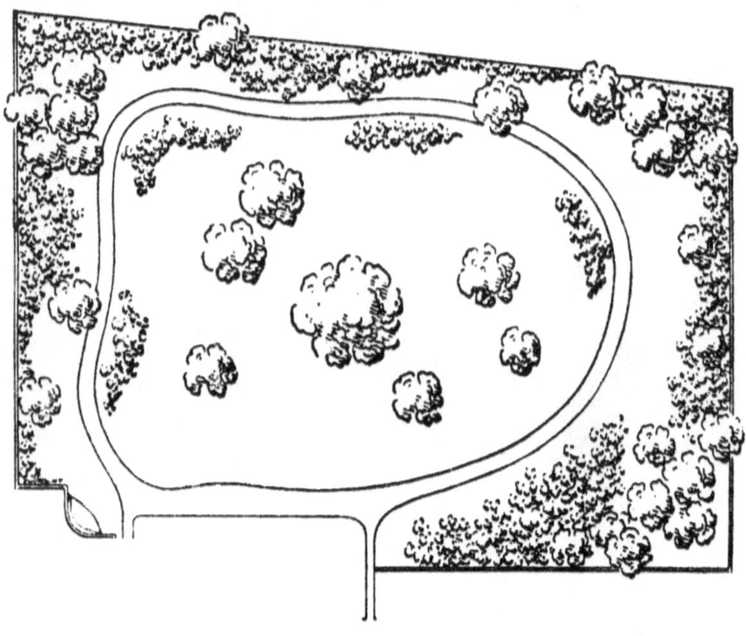

Let that first step be taken, and a second is all but
inevitable.
—*The Sunday at Home*

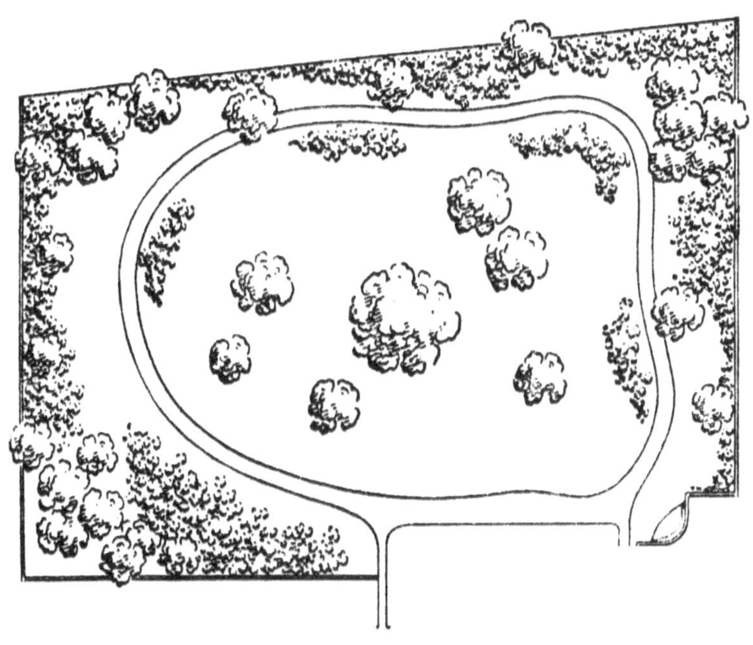

May your feet be saved from failing and your eyes
from tears.
—*Letters of St. Paulinus of Nola*

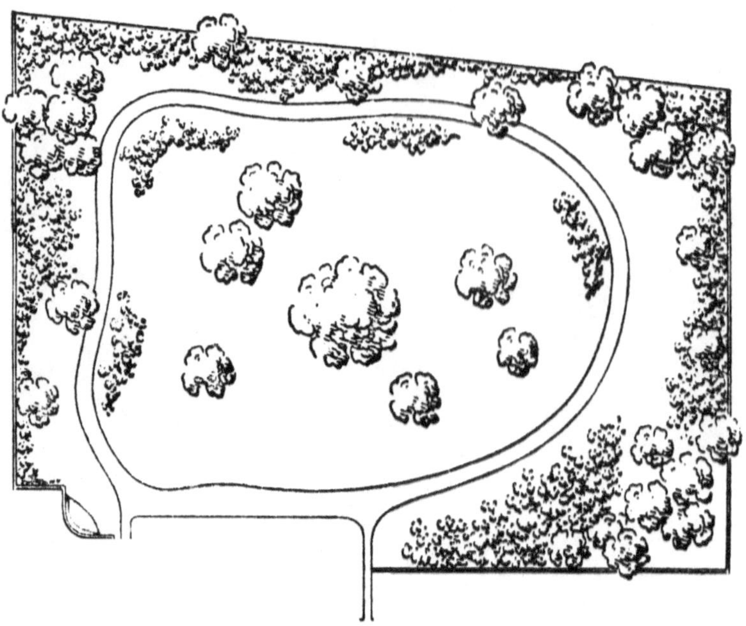

If the journey seems too difficult at times, if each step feels like your last, look back to see if the footprints behind are really yours.
—Phil Small, *On the Way to Here*

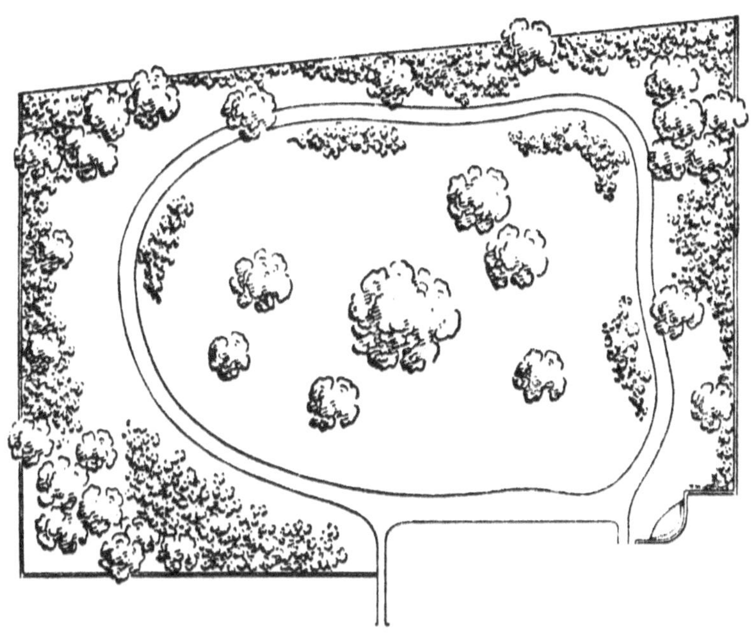

May your steps lead to wonders that delight your
heart.
—Barbara Moore, *Modern Guide to Energy Clearing*

You shall walk on your feet,
you shall not walk upside down.
—*The Egyptian Book of Going Forth By Day*

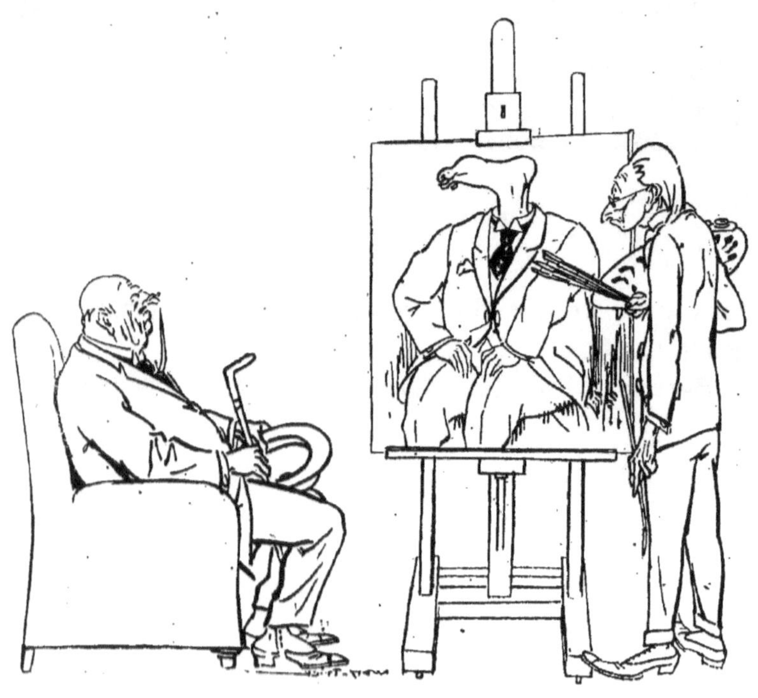

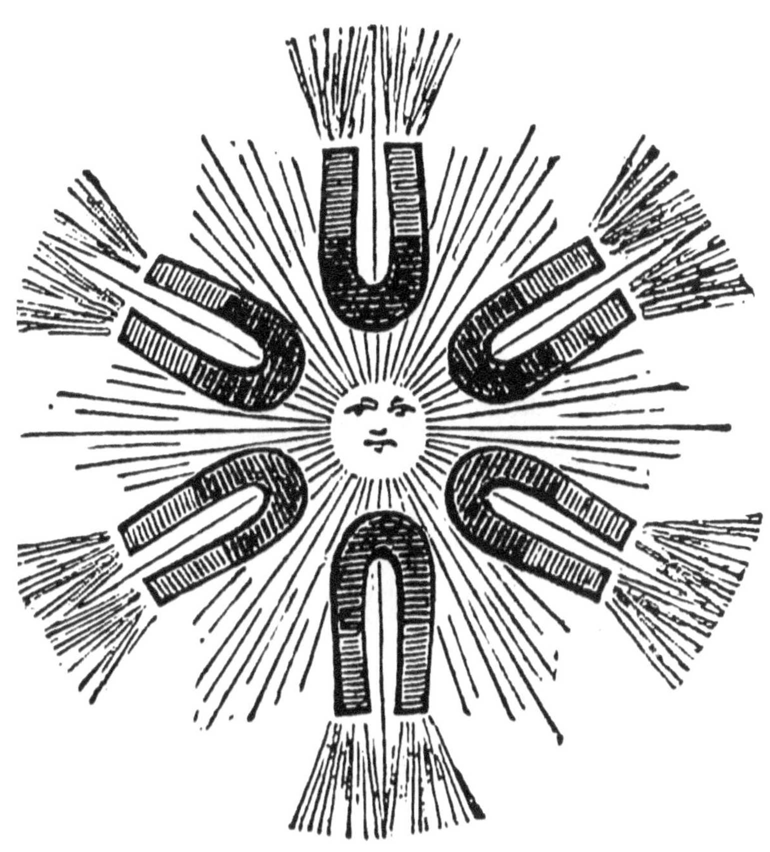

The Three Secrets to
Being Your Own Compass

When you come to a crossroads, the first secret of being your own compass is trusting your choice-making. "The universe will always present many options to you. As you learn to focus on what is important to you and only you, you will begin to see a clearer road. You will begin to trust your choices and choose the one prominent road of your life. Trust and be your own compass" (Alicja Bialasiewicz, *Never Fear Change*).

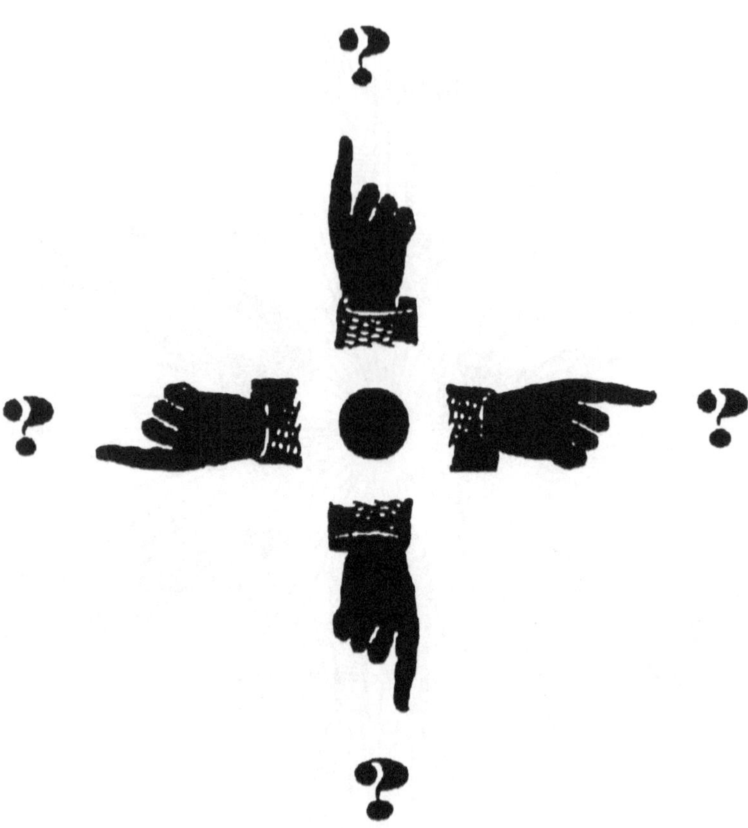

The second secret to being your own compass
is the practice of silence. Stop, listen, feel, breathe in,
and "be quiet enough to sense your own direction, to
hear the truth inside yourself, to know what is real,
to be your own compass. To be your own compass
is something we all have to be—no one can know
the right direction for another—we have to follow
our own truth" (Penelope Jewell, in her foreword to
Warrior of Truth by Ev Murray).

The third secret of being your own compass is being courageous enough to take the next step. "You've got to do it yourself. You've got to get out there, explore the world, be your own compass, and forge a road in life that is indicative of only one thing: yourself" (Mike Marriner & Nathan Gebhard, *Roadtrip Nation*).

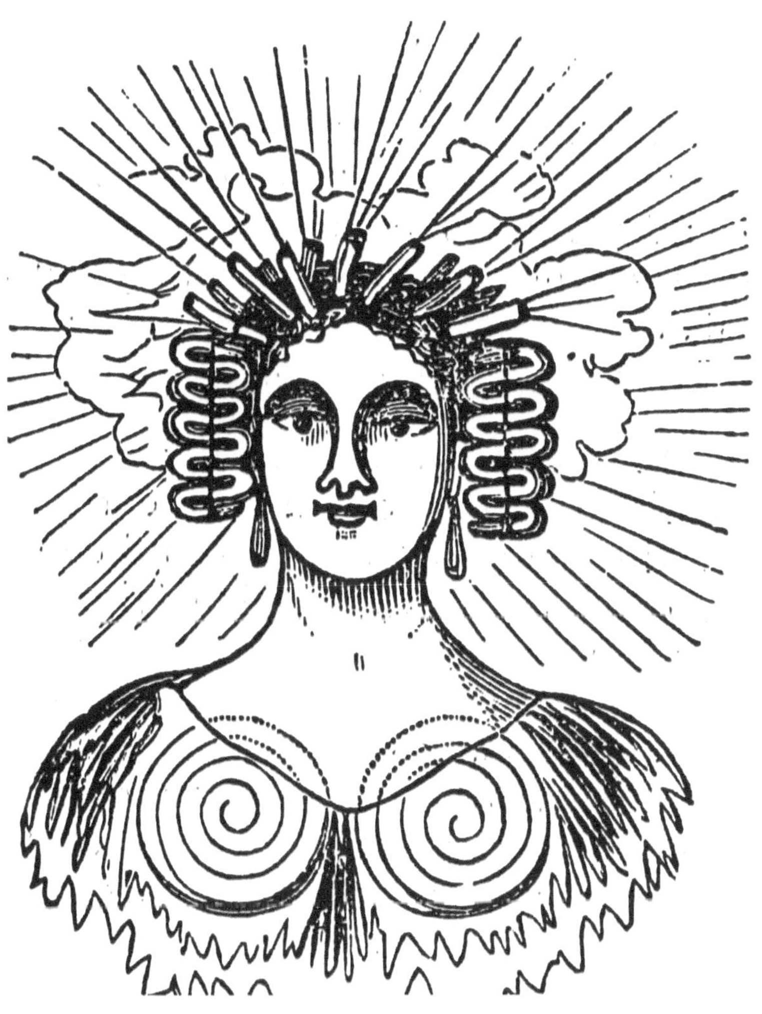

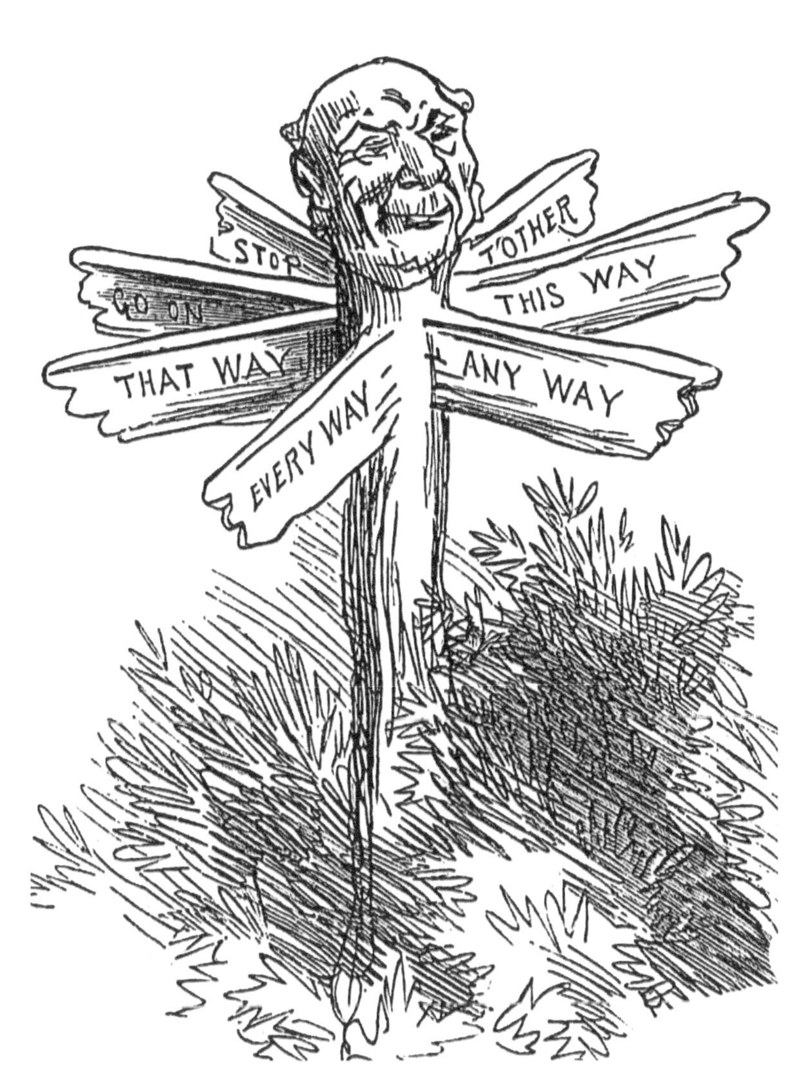
STOP
GO ON
THAT WAY
EVERY WAY
T'OTHER
THIS WAY
ANY WAY